SURVIVING YOUR DOCTORS

SURVIVING YOUR DOCTORS

Why the Medical System is Dangerous to Your Health and How to Get through it Alive

Richard S. Klein, M.D.

ROWMAN & LITTLEFIELD PUBLISHERS, INC.
Lanham • Boulder • New York • Toronto • Plymouth, UK

Published by Rowman & Littlefield Publishers, Inc.
A wholly owned subsidiary of The Rowman & Littlefield Publishing Group, Inc.
4501 Forbes Boulevard, Suite 200, Lanham, Maryland 20706
http://www.rowmanlittlefield.com

Estover Road, Plymouth PL6 7PY, United Kingdom

British Library Cataloguing in Publication Information Available

Library of Congress Cataloging-in-Publication Data

Klein, Richard S., 1938–
  Surviving your doctors : why the medical system is dangerous to your health
and how to get through it alive / Richard S. Klein, M.D.
      p. cm.
  Includes bibliographical references and index.
  ISBN 978-1-4422-0139-2 (cloth : alk. paper) — ISBN 978-1-4422-0141-5
(electronic)
  1. Medical errors—United States. 2. Medical care—United States. 3. Self-
care, Health. I. Title.
  R729.8K64 2010
  610.28'9—dc22   2009027238

∞ ™ The paper used in this publication meets the minimum requirements of
American National Standard for Information Sciences—Permanence of Paper
for Printed Library Materials, ANSI/NISO Z39.48-1992.

Printed in the United States of America

This book is dedicated to the memory of John and the thousands of Americans who needlessly die every week

CONTENTS

Foreword   ix

Acknowledgments   xi

Introduction   I

SECTION I: EVERYDAY MEDICAL AND HEALTH CONCERNS

I   Taking Control of Your Health Care: Or the Wisdom of
    Second and Third Opinions   7

2   Insurance Companies: Organized Crime or Just Bad Policies?   13

3   An Apple a Day: And Other Things to Protect Your Health
    When Visiting the Doctor's Office   25

4   Does Your Kid Really Need that Shot? Protecting Your
    Children in the System   57

5   The Pharmacy and Prescription Drugs: Or Beware of the
    Spoonful of Sugar that Helps the "Medicine" Go Down   67

6   Visiting the Emergency Room without Feeling Like a
    Bit-Player on a Television Drama   73

SECTION II: MAJOR DISEASES AND LONG-TERM ISSUES

7   A Real Heart-to-Heart About Cardiac Care   101

8   How to Handle the Big C from A to Z: Coping with
        Cancer Treatment   107

9   Baby Boom or Bust: How to Stroll through Maternity,
        Neonatal, and Fertility Issues   117

10 You Give Me Fever: Infection and Communicable Diseases   129

11 How to Maintain Some Sanity in the Mental Health System   139

SECTION III: THE HOSPITAL AND MAJOR PROCEDURES

12 Hospital Outpatient Visits and How to Make Sure You
        Actually Get Out!   149

13 Hospital Stays: As Dangerous as a War Zone?   157

14 Medical Tests and How to Avoid becoming a Lab Rat!   169

15 Major Surgeries: Or How to Make Sure You Still Have a
        Leg to Stand on Afterward!   177

SECTION IV: THE FUTURE OF MEDICINE

16 A Cure for the Medical System   191

Notes   203

Resources   213

Bibliography   217

Index   225

About the Author   235

FOREWORD

Richard Klein introduces the raison d'être for his latest work, *Surviving Your Doctors*, as providing a "basic training manual" to guide patients through the "medical minefield" that is the modern practice of medicine. His basic premise is that "at least 100,000 patients die in American hospitals because of malpractice," and the purpose of this book is nothing less than to immediately start saving "tens of thousands of lives a year" and "ultimately save millions more in generations to come."

The author's perspective reflects his 38 years in the medical profession, including the past 25 years that he spent "reviewing thousands of medical malpractice cases for plaintiffs (the injured) and frequently testifying against guilty physicians or ancillary health care providers." In New York, almost 70 percent of plaintiffs do not prevail in their lawsuits, and one wonders how many of them were perhaps "injured" by the medical system as opposed to their disease process. Despite the wonderful advances of our medical system and the care and diligence of the health care team, 77-year-old men presenting in abdominal crisis sometimes die from their disease process rather than errors in the medical care they received. Having said that, Dr. Klein is absolutely correct when he points out that as a society we need to promote an environment where health care providers can discuss errors and "near misses" in an open way, free from intimidation or repercussion. It is well known that one of the foundations of the extraordinary safety record of the airline industry alluded to in the book is the freedom that all members of the profession have to freely and openly discuss errors, without fear of reprisals. Medical conferences where "morbidity and mortality" can be discussed openly and candidly are critical for error prevention and have no place in discovery and the legal process.

Regardless of whether one agrees with Dr. Klein's perspective on the medical system as a whole, certainly his advice to individual patients is right on target. Patients should be aware of every medication they take and not blindly follow orders. We all need to be active participants in our own health care, both at the preventative level in our choice of lifestyles (healthy eating, avoiding cigarettes, regular exercise, etc.) and in our conversations and questioning of our doctors and nurses. When patients, physicians, nurses, hospital staff, and pharmacies all work together, optimal health care is provided, and we as patients have our best chance at cure. At my own hospital, there are multiple signs that prominently advise patients and their families to remind all of their caregivers to wash their hands. This may sound silly or obvious, but routine and regular hand washing is more effective than antibiotics in preventing infection, and this hospital policy may save lives. When it comes to health insurance companies, Dr. Klein's description is both Kafkaesque and correct, and his advice on selecting your insurance plan is right on.

The advice Dr. Klein offers to patients reflects a tremendous body of experience and is worth thinking about. His mantra, "being an active participant in one's health care is essential for survival," is a morsel worth savoring. And whether you ultimately agree with Dr. Klein or not, his views are thought provoking and, despite his stated intention, may indeed "shock and scare the reader." When it comes to our health, that may be an appropriate prescription.

Dr. Michael Rosenberg
Past-president, Medical Society of the State of New York

ACKNOWLEDGMENTS

This, my second book, required many hours of research and a lot of advice from my medical friends and colleagues. Robert Schwartz and Jacob Harris gave up hours of their free time to make sure that I got pediatrics and psychiatry (respectively) down correctly. I also thank my friends Janusz Rudnicki and Gino Bottino for their input in ob/gyn and oncology. I thank Michael Rosenberg, president of the New York State Medical Society, for his thoughtful words in the foreword. My wife, Caryn, has been at my side during all of the time that was committed to produce this work. And lastly, many thanks to my "writing coach" Derek Rydal, who was there any time that I got stuck or had a question.

INTRODUCTION

The malpractice crisis is malpractice (itself).

—Vice President Albert Gore, May 1993[1]

The problem is not a malpractice insurance crisis. Nor, contrary to popular mythology, is the problem a lawsuit crisis. The real crisis is the degree of malpractice itself.

—*Business Week*, August 3, 1987[2]

Every year at least 100,000 patients die in our American hospitals because of malpractice.[3] You might want to read that statistic again. It is more than the number of soldiers who died in the Korean and Vietnam wars combined.

Every year.

That is like having *300 jumbo jets crash* and kill everyone!

Every year!

Or one jumbo jet crashing *almost every day*!

And that figure doesn't represent those who are hurt or maimed, which is probably two to three times that number. And the price to these individuals, their families, and society at large is approximately $30 *billion annually*![4] The financial and human costs are staggering.

Out of the 800 million passengers who fly every year in the United States, on average 50 to 200 are killed in commercial air crashes.[5] If that figure were artificially raised to 100,000 people killed in crashes, the percentage of mishap would be low, but frightening. In comparison, there are 36 million admissions to the 5,700 hospitals in the United States annually and at least 100,000 people are killed by medical malpractice.[6] Certainly, this is a larger percentage than flying mishaps.

However, if jumbo jets started falling out of the sky like flies don't you think there would be an outcry or maybe an investigation? I think that we can say with certainty that the entire air travel industry would grind to a screeching halt and the whole world would become galvanized around the issue. But how often do you hear stories focusing on this medical crisis? How many politicians are speaking about it in Congress? How often does the president address the fact that more people die every year in medical mistakes than a total of *thirty* September 11 tragedies combined?

Instead, the news cycles are crammed with the latest celebrity news of who is dating whom and who is having whose baby.

Again, the question arises, where is the outcry about medical injuries and malpractice?

Surviving Your Doctors is that voice.

For too long, wrongful outcomes from substandard or negligent care have been swept under the rug. We hear from physicians complaining about the high cost of medical malpractice insurance. They besiege our political leaders regularly, asking that caps be placed on awards given to injured patients or their surviving family members. High insurance premiums have forced good doctors out of the medical business. Others have stopped performing high-risk procedures. And all of this has left patients with less access to advanced medicine and doctors who are less willing to really engage in an intimate way, the only way that can ultimately lead to better health care in the long run.[7]

Patients need to know what is really going on, and just like walking into a war zone, they need to know how to protect and defend themselves. In this book I provide the in-depth explanations, guidance, and directions that will be the basic training manual we all need to survive and, hopefully, even to thrive. This book will serve as a map of the medical minefield, designed to show you where to step, where to stop, how to walk around the danger, and how to get out alive. Filled with case studies (in all cases names are pseudonyms to protect patient identities), anecdotes, questionnaires, and checklists, this book will walk you through every major area of the medical world—from the doctor's office, through the pharmacy, to the labs, outpatient procedures, hospital stays, surgery, and the emergency room—giving you a clearer picture of how things really work, what the workers really think, what is really going on, and how to take back control of your health care destiny once and for all. If you take to heart what is in these pages, I believe it will be an invaluable tool in your wellness kit.

This book may not solve all the sociopolitical issues surrounding this silent pandemic, but it will prepare you to protect yourself against these needless medical mistakes. And maybe, if enough of us begin to speak up, our media and our leaders will begin to wake up to the number three killer in America—*the medical industry itself.*[8]

But the intention, and if I dare say, the mission, of this book is much more. It is nothing less than to immediately start saving tens of thousands of lives a year while laying the foundation for, and sparking a national dialogue about, our healthcare system that will ultimately save millions more lives in the generations to come.

I

EVERYDAY MEDICAL AND HEALTH CONCERNS

1

TAKING CONTROL OF YOUR HEALTH CARE: OR THE WISDOM OF SECOND AND THIRD OPINIONS

> Mankind has survived all catastrophes. It will also survive modern medicine.
>
> —Gerhard Kocher[1]

My friend John was an elderly Italian American who always wore a warm smile. He was one of my favorite patients. At 77, he was physically fit and still worked part time, fixing kitchen appliances. Every summer he would bring in large boxes of homegrown zucchini, basil, tomatoes, and anything else he could grow. He was proud of his farming ability.

One year I told him I was thinking about planting my own vegetable garden. The next day he showed up at my home with a shovel, asking my wife where I wanted to plant it. I was amazed and honored by his unasked-for generosity. Unfortunately, the ground that I had chosen was rock hard, not ever having been worked before, and we had to get a roto-tiller to turn the soil over. I am a city boy and living in the suburbs has been quite an education. I didn't even know how to grow a tomato when I first started gardening. And my knowledge of a roto-tiller was far less. When I picked it up at the rental office, they told me to "hold it back when I used it." They meant that I needed to put a little back pressure into it as it propelled forward. Instead, I took their advice to mean that I should pull it backward.

John, it turned out, knew less than I did about this contraption, despite his years of growing those wonderful vegetables. Together, we spent four hours and every fiber of muscle we had to drag that tiller backward, trying to till an area only twenty by twenty feet! We were dirty, sweaty, and exhausted when we returned it, only to find out that we had done it completely wrong. We felt like fools, of course. But we laughed about it every time John paid me a visit because of his chronic medical issues.

As is the procedure when I am off during a particular weekend, the answering service awakens me on Monday morning to inform me of any admissions to my service. John had been admitted late Sunday night with an acute abdomen. Often, when a close friend or patient gets sick, I get that adrenalin rush, becoming both anxious and revved up, as well as touched by sadness. I rushed to see my "tiller" buddy.

At 7 A.M., John was near death, his abdomen felt as hard as a diving board and his pulse was weak and thready, racing at 110 beats per minute. These were all sure signs that an abdominal organ had ruptured and acute peritonitis had set in. I quickly called the surgeon, who had admitted him five hours earlier. "Gosh," he said, "John's abdomen was soft and nontender when I left him." At the surgeon's request, while he rushed in, I called the operating room to prepare. I then went down to the emergency room and reviewed John's record.

Unfortunately, because of his initial intense pain he had been given an injection of meperidine (Demerol) just before the surgeon had arrived. Analgesics, especially narcotics, should never be given to anyone with an abdominal crisis until the exact nature of the complaint is known. The narcotic relaxes the abdominal muscles as it relieves the pain and tenderness, thereby hiding findings that an examining doctor needs for evaluation. In other words, the emergency room physician not only killed the chance for my friend to be properly diagnosed and treated in a timely manner, he killed my friend. This isn't an exaggeration. His error was the direct cause of why John died as they placed him on the operating table.

This book is dedicated to the memory of John and the other 90,000 patients in our American hospitals who die needlessly, every year, because of medical malpractice. As I mentioned in the Introduction, that is equivalent to 300 jumbo jets crashing and killing everyone on board every year. That is one jumbo jet crashing almost every day.

Surely, the medical world is not the safest place to be. My intention here is not to shock or scare you from ever entering a physician's or dentist's office again. Neither is it meant to discourage you from treatment in a hospital or emergency room. I have been a practicing physician in the fields of internal medicine and infectious diseases, as well as teacher at a medical school, for the past 38 years. For the past 25 years I have been reviewing thousands of medical malpractice cases for plaintiffs (the injured) and I frequently testify against guilty physicians or ancillary health care providers.

Both physicians and the public at large have to deal with the core problem. They have to acknowledge that medical malpractice occurs. I feel that it causes death and disability to an unfortunately large portion of our patients. This book is an attempt to educate both sides, with the goal of promoting open communication and dialogue.

Patients need to know how to navigate the mine fields of the medical world and how to involve themselves in their own care. No longer should you just swallow a pill handed to you by a nurse, or increasingly more common, by an aide. Knowing that one of the single most common causes of hospital negligence that occurs is from mistakes resulting in adverse drug reactions, you should ask what a pill is for and why it is actually needed.[2] It is probably more prudent to ask your physician to list all of the medications that you will be prescribed during your hospital stay. In this way, you will know which pills or injections were really designated for your body. All too often, a nurse will enter a room, ask you to turn over, and inject you with something that was intended for the patient in the next room.

Most of us older physicians know that effective open communication with our patients will lower the number of malpractice suits. That is because we talk to our patients and allow them to become a part of the treating team. We must, however, set up better guidelines to protect the safety of those in our care and to empower patients to become educated about their health care options.

Years ago I was crawling through a newly dug tunnel under Mount Moriah, sacred to both Jews and Muslims. One member of my group, crawling next to me, complained that he had dirtied his raincoat and that it was the only one that he had brought with him on this three-day, ambassador-level trip to Israel. I looked at him and realized that it was Sy Simms, well known because of his television ads for his clothing stores. Only someone in the clothing business would be upset about having only one raincoat with him! The Simms's slogan was "An educated consumer is our best customer."

I want you to be an educated medical consumer. I want you to be informed about what is really going on. I want you to be in control of your health care rather than placing it, through blind faith, into the hands of an industry that is simply not designed to have your best interests at heart most of the time. My hope is also that this book, together with you, the informed patient, will stimulate the medical licensing boards, as well as the medical societies and hospitals, to attack the medical malpractice problem as if we were threatened with a pandemic—which is really what it is. I feel that we, the medical practitioners, have to admit to the fact that we, albeit nonintentionally, sometimes injure people. Rather than worry about being sued, we should be able to talk to our patients when these departures from good standards of care exist. We should discuss them with our hospitals and make sure that the patients or their survivors are adequately compensated. But in order to make this movement happen, it is going to take you, the informed patient, to fully participate in your own health care.

In this high-tech world, any human endeavor can and will be associated with mistakes. Millions of accidents outside of medicine occur yearly. Just a few years ago, our government sent a billion dollar satellite into orbit that went entirely in the opposite direction intended. The technician mistakenly put in coordinates in metric instead of American standard values. We, as physicians, strive for perfection, but we have to understand that perfection cannot always happen. Perfection is impossible when we deal with so many facts and nuances. We make unintentional mistakes that, until now, we were taught to deny. We conjure up all sorts of excuses, blaming the laboratory, the x-ray department, the nurses. It reminds me of some of my patients who get fired from their jobs. I often hear someone say "the supervisor had it in for me" or something similar. It is rare to overcome one's denial, as I almost never hear someone admit to messing up. It seems that to me that we physicians never ask how did I contribute or how can I make sure that we, the medical community, don't do it again? If we do not admit that we caused the problem and speak up about it, how will the problem get fixed? Certainly not by capping medical malpractice insurance or lowering our insurance rates.

The health care crisis is multifactorial. It begins long before a patient ever engages a health care professional. It starts with the type of insurance or Medicare coverage that one has, if one is lucky enough to have insurance at all. But it certainly does not stop there. At every stage throughout your healing journey there are things you need to be aware of. Throughout the chapters of this book, I will take you, the patient (or potential patient), along with me as I see patients in my office, make my rounds, and send patients to radiology or the laboratory for testing. I will show you what could happen while you are in the emergency room or operating room if you are not properly informed. I will give the whole health care industry a "second opinion." And by preparing you, I will enable you to become your own best health care advocate every time you are treated within the health care industry.

2

INSURANCE COMPANIES: ORGANIZED CRIME OR JUST BAD POLICIES?

Financial ruin from medical bills is almost exclusively an American disease.

—Roul Turley[1]

THE STATE OF HEALTH INSURANCE

Contrary to what many Americans are told, and perhaps believe, we do not have the best health care or health care system in the world. According to the World Health Organization (WHO), our system is rated lower than most European countries, including the former eastern bloc countries of Poland and the Czech Republic.[2] People in those nations all have longer life spans than we do, and their infant and child mortality and morbidity rates are significantly less. Survival rates for breast and colon cancer seem to be better in these thirty-six other countries. It is true that people come from all over the world to obtain our expertise. This does support the argument that some of our institutions offer the best knowledge that money can buy. But this expertise is available in only 5 percent of our nation's hospitals. If you do not have the proper insurance or do not live anywhere near a particular medical institution, you may not get the care you need.[3] We have 50 million uninsured citizens who, study after study, get significantly lower standards of health care than the rest of us and who are a prime target of medical malpractice.[4]

Health care insurance companies are in existence to make money. On one hand, you cannot really blame them. They are, after all, for-profit companies that are legally bound to maximize shareholder value. It seems their need for profit is oftentimes in direct conflict with the patient's need for adequate and affordable coverage.[5] This is one of the main premises of Michael Moore's movie *Sicko*. In a very real sense, there is a dangerous conflict of interest here. That topic is beyond the scope of this book, however, but it is something you need to understand so that you can go into the insurance game with your eyes wide open. If we cannot solve this inherent conflict, you can at least be better prepared based on real-world knowledge of how the system works.

It seems to many as if insurance companies were in business merely to make a buck. Plain and simple. One way to reduce their liability, and therefore increase their potential profitability, is to cherry pick their future clients.[6] Many applicants for private insurance are either rejected because of some minimal abnormality found while reviewing their medical records or else they have riders placed on them that do not cover preexisting conditions.[7] These riders may be for a period of one to two years. If you have a chronic illness, you may not be eligible for coverage for that illness, or for any complication thereof, forever.

Some companies offer coverage in some geographic areas where there is a paucity of providers. I have cared for patients whose insurance company afforded access to most specialists, but they were literally in far away counties. I would have had to send a patient twenty or thirty miles away to a surgeon or hospital I didn't know.

Because of reimbursement rates declining every year as compared to the cost of doing business (i.e., inflation, raises for staff, and increases in rents and supplies), physicians have to see more patients, in the same time frame, as they previously did to offset these rising costs. I have seen firsthand that these pressures cause many physicians to take short cuts, and this can ultimately lead to greater inattentiveness. The only way a referring physician, such as myself, can get to know which specialist is going to take good or bad care of my patient is by either using him or her as a referral over a period of time or by getting feedback from my colleagues. If I am forced to send a patient to a distant specialist, it is going to be hit or miss. Not all specialists are great, just as not all baseball players become most valuable players. Understanding how your insurance company and doctor will deal with these issues can mean the difference between adequate care and excellent care and could have a significant impact on your future quality of life. It is that important that you should ask certain questions before selecting the right health care insurance.

Probably the most important question to ask is which hospitals are covered by the proposed insurance policy. I will discuss later how to pick the right hospital in your vicinity. The hospital setting is where most people are either injured or die as a result of medical malpractice, so ensuring you have the choice of a top-notch one could literally become a life or death decision. I am not trying to be melodramatic here. Remember those statistics? I do not want you to become one of them. For example, does the insurance policy cover specialty hospitals? Surprisingly, many companies don't. Is there coverage for complete annual physicals, in-vitro fertilization, bone marrow transplants, and so forth? This all may seem foreign to you now, but it is so critical in an emergent time of need. If you have the option, it is worth the time to sit down with a general agent, one who represents multiple insurance companies, rather than someone who represents only one.

Unfortunately, not all policies are the same, and you usually get what you pay for. The best options, such as being able to go to any specialist or obtain any test, without a primary care physician's (PCPs) referral, cost more. And with rising insurance rates and unstable economic times, not everyone can afford more. It seems as if some insurance companies actually reward PCPs for not overusing specialists or for not ordering a lot of computed tomography (CT) scans and magnetic resonance images (MRIs).[8] Did you catch that? It appears that doctors are often rewarded for not rendering, in some cases, the best and most effective medical treatment possible![9] The Cigna Insurance Company recently settled an agreement with the New York State attorney general Andrew Cuomo. Cigna and other insurance companies (Aetna for one) were making lists of their preferred physicians, whom they were recommending to their insured clients.[10] They also were making similar settlement deals with the attorney general. These providers were chosen, according to the statement by Cuomo, by the amount of money they saved the company. That is, their use of outside services, such as CT, MRI, and specialist referrals, was less than their peers'. It appears that they are rewarded for the lower cost to health maintenance organizations (HMOs) regardless of their talent. They were not chosen because they were the best physicians with the best outcomes. If that sounds like the exact opposite of what doctors are supposed to do, you're not crazy—it is! But that is the system to which many people are subjected. Bottom line, many insurance companies make it almost impossible to get permission to send a patient for a special test, a test that really could have a significant impact on the patient's health and the rest of his or her life.

I have had sick patients (who were not really categorized as emergencies) come in late in the afternoon with a diagnosis that could only be determined by an MRI or CT scan. Unfortunately, in many cases, the authorization department of their respective insurance carriers is closed at 3 P.M. Obviously, permission for the requested test would now have to wait until the next day, at minimum. With the average insurance company it takes 24 hours for the request to go through and, even after approval, it takes at least a week to schedule the test. This is certainly problematic for the patient, but it is also frustrating for the physician. Here the physician has a sick patient, but the patient is not quite sick enough to wait in the emergency room for hours to obtain the test at the hospital. How many patients have been sent home without the necessary tests for this reason and ended up with serious complications as a result? The answer is too many. Kelly rightfully went to her gynecologist after experiencing left lower abdominal pain. An ultrasound of her pelvis revealed some fluid in her cul-de-sac, a sign of a ruptured cyst. She was sent home with some analgesics and told it would shortly pass. The pain intensified and she saw me at about 4 P.M., two days later. Well, her pain seemed more like diverticulitis (an inflammation of an out pouching of her large intestine), and although she was not very ill, making the diagnosis required a CT scan. Her insurance company was closed for the afternoon, and so I treated her with the proper antibiotics and she gradually improved. It took two weeks to get approval for the test and by that time, her symptoms as well as her test (CT) were normal. Did I know for certain that her diagnosis was correct? If the symptoms recur in the future, will I have hard evidence of what she did have? The answer to both those questions is no, and that is not right.

To give you a better idea of just how out of whack and wasteful the insurance tangle has made the system, think about this: most physicians' offices employ at least one dedicated, full-time person, who spends eight hours a day phoning for permission (a referral) to send a patient to a specialist or for a special test. The employee does not earn *any* money for the physician, such as a nurse who gives an injection, nor does the employee help in the flow and efficiency of the office (such as a bookkeeper or typ-ist). The employee just sits there, day in and day out, fighting for patients' rights. And it really is a fight.

The procedure usually starts by the employee calling the assigned insur-ance carrier's telephone number. This is usually busy, as there are a lot of physicians' offices calling for referrals or permission to help their patients. When the call is finally answered, the employee is kept on hold for five to ten minutes. A receptionist or administrative advisor at the other end (not a nurse or physician) then takes all the information. If the patient does not meet certain "criteria" on the basic questionnaire, the test or service can be denied. Not denied by an informed doctor, or denied by a physician who has actually met or examined the patient, but denied by a receptionist working from a rule book!

The next step is for a request to speak to the nurse, who usually will call back within a few hours. If that step does not get the proper permission, the insurance company's physician is requested, and that can take four to six hours for a return call. On and on it goes—where it stops, only the insurance company knows.

The basic criteria are determined by a medical staff paid by the insur-ance company, and they are very stringent. Remember that insurance companies are in business to make money and, it seems, to discourage outside physicians, such as myself, from ordering tests. For example, I may have an overweight male smoker, who is 30 years of age and whose father died of a coronary infarction at the age of 35 or 40. Unusual? No. Many physicians see a few patients a year with similar stories. Wouldn't it be good to find beginning symptoms of heart disease early in one of these young men, to treat it, and prevent similar deaths that their parents had? Try to get permission from an insurance company for a stress test for a 30-year-old! "Are there any symptoms," you'll be asked. "Are there any abnor-malities on their electrocardiograms?" "Does it make good sense to do the test?" To the practicing physician it sure does. To the insurance company, the cost of screening all of these young men with stress tests far outweighs the benefit of saving a few patients. I can hear some of you saying, "But wait, that overweight smoker should take some responsibility for himself!" To which I would absolutely agree. But in the meantime, while he is sitting in my office two puffs away from a cardiac arrest, do I just let him die? Be-sides, there are hereditary factors that are not considered by the insurance company. There was a marathon runner by the name of Jim Fixx , who died at the age of 52, due to a heart attack. Everyone was stunned at his death because he was in such good shape, until they learned that his dad, who wasn't an athlete, died in a similar manner at the age of 35.

Again, it cannot be overstated that insurance companies are in the business of making money. Their medical staffs are often adequately paid, salaried physicians, some of whom have dropped out of mainstream medicine perhaps because of their own inabilities.[11] I know of two physicians who were removed from my local hospital's staff (that is, they lost their privileges) because they did not meet the normal levels of standard of care. These physicians took up positions in two different insurance companies. Another friend of mine, a surgeon, just couldn't stay busy enough to keep up with his overhead. He too left his practice and joined the ranks of an HMO. He now makes decisions all day on nonsurgical issues, such as whether permission should be given for an internist to order a stress test on a particular patient. I am told that some receive an annual bonus of up to 20 percent of their salaries.[12] I have also been told by two physician headhunters that this bonus has something to do with meeting established goals, usually financial in nature. They do not usually understand the nuances of the "art of medicine" and therefore are stuck within the rigid guidelines that they themselves have devised. My answer to an insurance company's denial is often "Can your (the insurance company physician's) conscience really live with that decision?" These insurance company "doctors" are making life-and-death decisions on patients they have never examined, let alone even seen. Their job is to keep the money in the company. At best, the above-described procedure is agonizing, costly to the physician's staff time, and conducive to just letting the test go. The type of policy that requires this amount of phone calling is one of the least expensive to the patient. And it is not uncommon for employers to offer this less expensive insurance to their employees because of the money it saves them. I recently examined a 50-year-old man who had a cough for a few weeks. Henry admitted to being a heavy smoker for 30-some-odd years. I asked my secretary to obtain permission for a baseline CT scan of his lungs. Not an unusual request, as Henry was a prime contender for lung cancer. I wasn't suspecting that disease, but it is very helpful to have such a baseline study. Sure enough, Friday morning, we received a written denial from his insurance carrier. Unfortunately, that same evening, Henry started coughing up blood, winding up in the local emergency room. Yes, an emergency CT revealed that he not only had lung cancer, but it had spread to the covering of his heart.

Recent political ads against universal health care are scary by suggesting that government bureaucrats will be put between you and your doctor. The reality is that we already have bureaucrats placed between you and your physician. They just happen to work to save money for the insurance companies.

Another major problem with insurance coverage is the limitation of medications a physician can order. Most insurance companies arrange financial deals with a pharmaceutical house, obtaining medicines at a cheaper rate for each disease. I had a patient on a cholesterol lowering medicine, atorvastatin (Lipitor). The next year, his insurance company said they would only pay for older, less used medicines or, perhaps, for a drug called simvastatin (Zocor). To save the patient from a larger copay, I ordered the simvastatin (there is a pharmacological difference between atorvastatin and simvastatin). The next year, the same insurance company must have made a better deal with the makers of atorvastatin again, because now they wanted us to switch back to this drug. Multiply that by many drugs for many diseases for each health insurance company—and add to it all the calls to get approval on tests—and you start to get a picture of how many hours at a busy physician's office are wasted by keeping up with the ever-unraveling red tape of insurance companies. How much better service, at more economical prices, do you think doctors could provide if they did not have to waste endless hours in this bureaucratic quagmire? If it is confusing for the physician, who lives with it daily, imagine how confusing it is for a patient who has to change medicines every year or two (not out of medical necessity, but out of insurance company politics and profit).

And the problems don't stop there. There are many newer and expensive medicines that have to be precertified. Just like trying to obtain permission for an MRI or CT scan, my secretary has to spend fifteen to thirty minutes to obtain permission for a patient to get a particular medicine. What is the underlying agenda behind this new obstacle course the insurance company has created? It often seems to us practicing physicians that it is to wear the doctors down so that they will give up, give in, and just accept the older, less effective, and, of course, cheaper therapy. What does all this have to do with the job of medicine, which is to get you better, quicker? Absolutely nothing! In fact, the result is all too often quite the opposite. Of course, the more expensive insurance policies allow the patient to get any test, see any specialist, and obtain any medication without the above hassle. But it is also no coincidence that the people who can afford more expensive insurance are often also able to afford better food, housing, hygiene, health clubs, and an overall healthier lifestyle, and therefore they tend to need health care less than those who cannot afford to get it and whose living conditions make them more prone to medical problems. And that is exactly what the insurance companies are banking on.

According to a November 3, 2008, *New York Times* editorial, women are often gouged on health insurance costs. "As tens of thousands of workers lose their jobs and their group health insurance, in a worsening economy, they will have to scramble to find affordable insurance policies in the open market. The problems will be particularly acute for women, who often pay far higher premiums than men for the same health coverage, if they can get coverage at all."[13] In a recent report by the National Women's Law Center, these inequities in the health insurance market were described in detail.[14] Federal antidiscrimination laws usually protect women who are covered by their employers' group policy. However, states regulate the market for individually bought policies, and most offer women little, if any, protection against discrimination. New York is a notable exception. Women can wind up paying hundreds of dollars a year more than men for identical coverage. Analyzing 3,500 individual health insurance plans found that insurers charged 40-year-old women anywhere from 4 percent to 48 percent more than they charged men of similar age. Also disclosed was the fact that in some states, insurers are allowed to reject applicants for reasons that effectively exclude many women, such as having had a Caesarean section or surviving domestic violence, and that the vast majority of these individual policies do not cover maternity care. Of course, the insurance industry justifies charging higher premiums on actuarial grounds because they say that women between the ages of 19 and 55 make greater use of health care services than do men. Women are more likely to have chronic conditions requiring ongoing treatment, they say, plus women are more likely to take prescription medications on a regular basis. Of course that is no explanation for the fact that one company charges 40-year-old women 140 percent more than men and another company only charges 15 percent more. Insurance companies used to charge higher premiums based on race, using the same actuarial argument. This practice has since been stopped. But remember, insurance companies are there to make money.

MEDICARE

When senior citizens approach age 65, they are entitled to Medicare. Initially, when Medicare first was introduced, in the late 1960s, most physicians were up in arms. As it was, Medicare became a very decent form of socialized medicine for the elderly. It allowed for specialists and testing without referrals or insurance company permission. Medicare covered the noninsured and many needy elderly people. Although the reimbursements for physicians were significantly lower than most third party payers at the time, the government paid on time. And because there was no calling needed for referrals or permission for tests, these patients reduced additional time and expenses to the doctor, ultimately making them cost-effective to treat.

Over the years, however, our government has gone into trillions of dollars of debt (for nonmedical reasons). And with the ever-rising cost of health care, something had to give. Now the elderly, who need preventive health care the most, suffer if they have Medicare alone. Annual physical examinations, with electrocardiograms, chest x-rays, blood screening, bone densities, and other test are denied to Medicare recipients.[15] The elderly have to have an illness or a symptom to obtain a test. With the news media and medical experts touting the benefits of early detection for cancers, heart disease, diabetes, and other diseases, doesn't it make sense that the group of people most likely to get these diseases should have better access to screening? Ironically, Medicare even states that the elderly should have annual physicals, but they won't pay for it. The government simply cannot afford it. We read daily that there are more and more cutbacks from Medicare to physicians and hospitals. Teaching hospitals are being forced to cut back on staff, resident and intern training programs, as well as research, which is resulting in poorer care today and certainly in poorer care for tomorrow.

One of the reasons I wrote this book is to make all of us more informed, proactive citizens when it comes to our own health care and our ailing health care system. Understanding the connection between the insurance crisis and the malpractice epidemic is a big part of that. The fact is that it costs us, the taxpayers, billions of dollars annually to pay for the medical malpractice that rains down upon us every year. Instead of caring for the medically injured, maimed, or dying as a result of malpractice, imagine if that money were used for comprehensive health care for all of our citizens?

So what is the connection between this lack of adequate insurance coverage for Americans—especially the elderly—and the growing government debt and medical crisis we are facing? Studies show that most Medicare recipients cannot afford secondary health insurance, which is necessary to pay the 20 percent of a bill not covered by Medicare. Furthermore, prescription drug coverage for the average elderly American is almost nonexistent. Medicines and treatments cost many elderly hundreds of dollars monthly. If, because of a lack of secondary insurance and prescription coverage, they cannot afford their medicines to keep them in "medical balance," these recipients become much sicker, are hospitalized on a more frequent basis, and add massive additional costs to the mounting financial burden, straining the already overwhelmed health care system. Similar to Russian roulette, the more and more one is admitted into a hospital, the greater the odds become that someone will be exposed to medical malpractice.[16]

YOUR ROLE

This is a vicious cycle that won't magically cure itself. The current system doesn't work. The lack of adequate health care coverage and the bureaucratic nightmare of insurance companies lead to massive waste, inefficiencies, ineffectiveness, and doctors and other health practitioners becoming overstressed. This leads to inattentiveness, medical errors, increased malpractice, and more sick and dying patients. Over and over. We either do something about it, or eventually the system will collapse completely under its own weight and deteriorating structures.

So what can you do about this? The rest of this book will certainly address that. But to begin with you must be your own best health care advocate. You must take back your health destiny. Of course that means taking the best care of yourself as possible. But it also means asking questions—lots of questions—of your insurance provider and medical practitioner. It means writing to your political representatives and demanding change in these policies. It means becoming a more informed, more active citizen in this area.

If you have options regarding the type of health insurance you choose, do the research to find out exactly what they provide and what doctors think about them. If you cannot afford to get a better health insurance provider, then use the information in this book to take control of your experience through the health care system, thereby ensuring much better care. If you have no insurance at all, do whatever you can to get it—even if it is only catastrophic coverage—and then take the best care of yourself that you possibly can. That means adopting a healthy diet and exercise program. In the end, that is your best insurance policy.

PRESCRIPTION

- Obtain some protection with health insurance and prescription coverage. If you are young and healthy, catastrophes do happen but are less likely. If you cannot afford full coverage or your employer doesn't supply insurance, at least obtain catastrophic coverage. This is bare bones insurance that just covers expensive emergencies such as an acute appendicitis or sports-related joint injury, requiring a lot of surgery.
- If you are out of work or in school or work at a company that does not provide health insurance, try to find a part-time job with a company that makes coverage available to even part-time workers. Currently, companies such as Starbucks, JC Penney, Target, Nike, and Nordstrom, just to name a few, offer such access.[17] Make sure that your coverage will pay for the hospital of your choice, as well as for your PCP and his or her team of specialists—anesthesiologists, radiologists, and specialized hospitals in your vicinity.
- Get to know a general life and health insurance agency. Some are really knowledgeable and can get you in and out of some insurance companies for a specific illness. Your present insurance company may not cover fertility or perhaps an admission into a special cancer care hospital. It is possible to temporarily change your present coverage to help pay for your specific problem.
- Take care of yourself; eat a healthy diet and exercise regularly. Good food and a healthy lifestyle are your best medicine!

3

AN APPLE A DAY:
AND OTHER THINGS TO PROTECT
YOUR HEALTH WHEN VISITING
THE DOCTOR'S OFFICE

The doctor is often more to be feared than the disease.

—French Proverb[1]

So here you are, rushing into your doctor's appointment, maybe filled with anxiety, your mind swirling with fears of illness, painful treatments, and a lifetime of prescriptions. You are not sure what to say or what to do, and you are stressed because you have to get back to work before lunch is over. Ironically, the lack of a healthy lunch and the increased stress are both bad for your health!

But this time it is going to be different. This time I am going to be with you. Well, not literally of course, but through these pages. And when we are done with our little virtual tour, you are going to know how to be there for yourself more than you have ever been before. So, take a breath and step inside the doctor's office with me.

Most patients find going to a physician's office very stressful but obviously necessary. Rule number one is to be on time even though your physician may not be (we will deal with doctor tardiness later). Calling to say you are stuck in traffic is courteous. Getting stuck more than once . . . not so courteous. Neither should you show up two hours early, thinking that you will get squeezed in and out more quickly. Office staff hate that. (Remember all the time they waste on insurance company issues? They also do not want to spend more time playing musical doctor appointments with the schedule.) Be clean and do not smell. I am not being humorous here. Doctors and medical practitioners are people, too. And they do not like spending a lot of time with people who smell! If you are a smoker, pop a breath mint; if you are a construction worker, put on some deodorant. This may sound trite or superficial, but the fact is, if you smell, you are much more likely to get a less-than-thorough examination, at least from me. Years ago, I cared for a retired New York City police sergeant. He did not like people and had decided to live in a dilapidated house, in the woods, which did not have hot water. But worse than that, he lived with thirty or forty cats. Jim was a good soul and could intelligently discuss his 401K and all of his investments. But there was no way I was going to go anywhere near him. I couldn't get past my nose. Often he was sent home to find someone with a shower he could use before I would examine him. I also have a few chain smokers in my practice whose breath and overall odor were unbearable. I have had to send them off to the showers as well. I told one patient that he smelled so terrible he would have to go home and change. I didn't promise you that these tips would be pleasant, but I do promise you that if you follow them you will increase your chances of better care. By the way, I am not implying that you smell, so please don't take this personally.

Upon arrival, be smiling and cheerful even if you feel terrible. Treat everyone with kindness and respect. I know you are the client, you are the patient, you are paying their bills, and you should not have to do any of this. But all that really matters right now is that you don't end up on the "life is too short list," so that you can increase your chances of living a longer life! The fact is, no one likes a grumpy person and oftentimes doctors' offices' staff aren't taking into account the fact that you are acting out because you feel terrible or afraid. They just see one more problem patient and start watching the clock, waiting to go home. What is worse, if you act really rude you may wind up at the *end* of the patient list instead of at your allotted time slot. Yeah, they could do that to you. Don't give them a reason. It is not fair, it is not just. But it is the reality of it. One of my secretaries has a sign on her desk that states: "I can only please one person a day and today isn't your day. Tomorrow doesn't look to promising either."

Upon arrival, this is the opportunity to inform the front office of any demographic (insurance, address, name) changes. Choose an office worker whom you know or one you can identify by name (name tag). If you are waiting a long time, quietly ask some fellow patients around you when their appointments were. And if your wait extends even further or you are running late for another appointment, kindly explain your situation to the receptionist. Rarely, your chart may have been placed out of order or misplaced. However, your long wait is probably because of the doctor. Above all, don't take your anger out on the staff. It is the doctor who is usually keeping you waiting, not the staff. And the staff's job is to protect the doctors so they can do their job. That is what the staff are being paid for. Let's be honest, the doctor always wants to look good.

Finally, you are allowed into the inner office. You take a breath and, on your walk through the door, you reflect on your journey here: You fought lunch hour traffic, wolfed something down that only barely resembled food or skipped lunch altogether, you sped and rolled through a stop sign, risking a ticket and traffic school. And you did all of that so you could be kept waiting. The nerve! You are sick, you are angry, and that pretty woman with the blond hair sure didn't have to wait long! Just keep breathing, and put all that aside. There is an old medical adage that says that you shouldn't show your frustration to your neurosurgeon just before you are wheeled into the operating room for brain surgery. Similarly, try to refrain from complaining to your doctor about waiting too long. It is either part of his or her personality, or it is a symptom of the overburdened system. Either way, complaining won't help you and could, possibly, lead to inattentiveness that could hurt you. If it is really a problem that the appointments are always late, make an issue of it after your appointment. And if it does not resolve itself or you find the doctor treating you with less than excellent care, maybe it is time to find a new doctor.

Right now you have to concentrate on your reason for being there. Doctors can be intimidating. We like to think we are in control most of the time (even though we really are not), but when it comes to medicine—one of the most important issues in our life—most people become almost totally dependent on someone else. I say almost because, unlike years ago, you are now going to take an active role in your health care. With this book as a guide, you will now Google your symptoms, research the doctor or hospital, and have an idea of what is wrong and what testing should be done.

But first you have to overcome your anxiety about the doctor and your medical problem. Having fear of suffering from a serious disease intimidates you and keeps you from properly communicating with your doctor. Your doctor, on the other hand, is probably thinking with a clear head but is very busy. Physicians have lots of pressure on them and must hone their skills of communication to obtain their fullest concentration, at least in a perfect medical world. The reality is that many physicians do not hone their communication skills and are not thinking about how your fear is preventing you from expressing your symptoms and needs clearly. That is where you come in. That is why *you* have to take control. If this were a dance, this is where you would take the lead.

In my first book, *From Anecdote to Antidote*, I tried to demystify the current doctor-patient relationship. Patients would place their physicians on a pedestal of awe. Now I certainly like being idolized and it does well for my ego. However, physicians are regular people who take out the garbage, go shopping, and certainly make mistakes, just as all of us do. There has to be an easing of the trepidation I see in my patients' eyes as I consult with them for the first time. Putting me on a pedestal influences a patient's behavior while we discuss such important things as their medical history, weight, allergies, past medical procedures, and so forth. I cannot tell you how many second opinions I have given, often in complete reversal of a previous doctor's diagnosis, that could have been easily avoided if the patients had simply been more honest and less intimidated by their doctors during their initial consultation.

I can understand the sense of intimidation. Sometimes people feel uncomfortable or insecure around someone who may have had a more extensive education than they have. And, as in any human situation, there is the issue of "power." Think of it: you are entrusting your health and well-being into the hands of someone who (in most cases) went to school for an additional eight years after college and regularly cut into corpses as practice for tending to your health care needs. On top of which, you are sitting there in his or her office, on his or her turf, in a paper dress, with your backside hanging out. You will hear this from me time and again, the old way of looking at your physician has to be replaced by the viewpoint of the new, empowered patient. Talking up to your doctor puts you at a disadvantage where you really should be talking to your physician as an equal. Yes, he or she went to medical school and deserves to be respected for his or her knowledge. But that is where it ends. You are part of the new "treating team." You have to be empowered to look up everything and question, question, question your doctor. We make mistakes all of the time. My earlier book also dealt with doctors talking in "doctorese," which I will discuss later. Another issue that threatens the lives of patients is fear.

Fear of having a particular disease can oftentimes prevent patients from even seeing their doctors. There have been innumerable times, after examining a woman and finding a breast lump, I would ask if a patient knew there was a lump there. Most often the answer is yes, saying "I figured if you didn't find the lump then nothing was wrong."

The most important thing right now is being heard. You want to be able to communicate to your physician and have him or her listen to your complaints. Eye contact is very important. However, there should be some concern in your voice, which will get your doctor's attention. Paying him or her a compliment doesn't hurt either. There goes my ego.

It is the same ritual every three months. Michael comes in to see me quarterly for his multiple medical ailments. As I walk into his exam room, he presents me with a neatly typewritten note. On the top of the page are listed his medications and doses. Next are written any visits with other physicians, reasons for these visits, and the physicians' recommendations. Then he lists the reasons for this day's visit (check his blood pressure, any new symptoms or complaints, etc.) and a list of needed prescription refills. Since Michael works for the city, the last typed request is for a note proving that he was actually at the doctor's office that day. In our complex, hectic medical world, this is perfection.

We then discuss everything on his list in a quick and orderly fashion. There is still time to talk about his job, our families, and world happenings. That is how streamlined an "office visit template" can—and should—be. And that is what I want you to do when you see your doctor.

I always encourage my patients to write lists similar to this template and then bring it with them! One important point, never wait until your doctor is leaving the room on his or her way to the next patient to ask an important question. Your doctor's mindset is already finished with you and his or her thoughts are on the patient in the next room. That list that you so thoughtfully filled out and brought in should have covered that important question right up front. If you carry a PDA, BlackBerry, or whatever the latest planner/phone gadget is, you can keep it on there. I know I am starting to sound like a broken record, but being an active participant in one's health care is essential for survival. Furthermore, if you anticipate that there will be serious or deep discussions regarding a serious illness, bring an advocate. Once a patient hears the words "you have cancer," that patient will not hear another word for a while. Therefore, bringing a prepared advocate is important. Someone will have to be asking the right questions and writing down the answers. That surrogate will be calmer and perhaps he or she should bring a tape recorder as well as pencil and paper.

Just as important as being heard by your doctor is being proactive in the maintenance of your own health, which will also add strength to your voice. We are just as responsible as our physicians for our own health care, and so we must know as much as we can and must stay as informed as we can about the issues that relate to our health. You and only you are the best barometer of the goings-on in your own body. You know best when you feel normal and when you do not. But a doctor is almost always the best source of help if, and when, something does go wrong. And though our skills are many (if I do say so myself), we are not mind readers. We cannot just look at you and tell what you are thinking, what is bothering you, and what exactly is wrong. So you should never be afraid to ask your doctor a so-called stupid question, make a so-called dumb suggestion, or offer an observation that seems obvious. Do not hesitate to share any information that you have discovered, hunches you may have, or information you have heard about relevant health issues with your doctor. We, as physicians, certainly do not know everything.

As difficult as it is to suffer with a malady, or even the fear of one, it is more difficult to suffer in fear of the unknown. It is an unfortunate fact of life that disease happens. Fortunately, many diseases are curable if found early. If you take a positive approach to disease and are open with your doctor, you have a much higher chance of being one of the fortunate to be cured. You may or may not open the door—and your doctor's eyes—to a new avenue of treatment, but you will demonstrate your own level of commitment to your own health (something doctors appreciate and welcome), and that will go a long way to livening up those dry, clinical conversations.

After you go over your list of complaints, expect to be put through the regular routine examination, having your vital signs checked (temperature, blood pressure, pulse, respiration rate, and weight). Make sure the technician or nurse actually measures all of these values, instead of just asking "How much do you weigh?" More than likely, there will be a significant difference between what you think you weigh and what the scale actually says.

I once testified against an orthopedic surgeon who missed a serious wound infection in a patient. One of the complaints was that he never took the patient's temperature in all of the patient's post-op office visits. How could he know if the patient had a fever if he did not measure for one? His defense was that his staff never kept a thermometer in the office because they never needed one. He was serious.

In training, we internists used to chuckle because all surgeons believed their patients never got infected. It is ironic because you have to sign a consent form for any surgery and near the top of the list of informed complications you will find the word infection. One of the common causes of medical malpractice is the lack of recognition that a serious underlying infection is present.[2]

Weight is one of the most important vital signs. Fluctuations can be a valuable diagnostic tool. Weight loss without being on a diet can suggest endocrine disorders (such as an overactive thyroid gland or diabetes), cancers, and more commonly, anxiety and stress. Unexplained weight gain could also suggest endocrine disorders, such as underactive thyroid, water retention, congestive heart failure, organ failure (kidney, liver), poor peripheral circulation, massive tumor growth (rare), and most commonly (and, interestingly, the hardest one to accept for some people) unknowingly eating and drinking more calories than one should. I always find it amusing when, after an extensive negative workup for weight gain, so many patients will deny that it was their fault. Your doctor should do as thorough a history as possible. More than 90 percent of diagnoses are made just by the story you tell and the facts drawn out of you by asking the right questions. Physicians are taught to use open-ended questions versus closed-ended questions. A closed-ended question, such as "You never had that happen in a car?", is usually intimidating and often causes people to agree with the doctor, versus a more opened question, such as "Did it ever happen in a car?", which allows people to offer their own response. "No, it never happened in a car" is easier for a patient to respond to because it does not challenge what the doctor is saying. I want you to always challenge your doctor and to always be prepared to question, yes, question and question again.

We are taught to do physical examinations by the organ system. Lungs belong to the respiratory system and therefore the respiratory system is examined apart from the gastrointestinal system. Similarly, the neurological examination is done separately from anything relating to cardiology. So the question you must ask is: Were all of the parts of your body that are involved in your complaint examined? If you had a sore throat, were your throat, ears, nose, thyroid, as well as the glands under your neck examined?

If there were swollen glands, were the ones behind your ears, under your armpits, and in your groin examined? Presently, you may not know what body parts are involved in your particular complaints. That is understandable. You did not go to medical school. But that does not stop you from doing a little research online before going in. And it certainly does not stop you from asking your doctor: "What organs and functions are involved in (fill in your complaint)?" Then, you need to ask the doctor to check all those areas.

After the examination, your physician will usually (though not always) have your diagnosis and will suggest some testing to confirm or rule out possible diseases or disorders. It may be a simple urine test (no, you do not have to go home and study for a urine test), a complete blood count, or a scan of some kind. Once all the tests are in, the doctor (hopefully) will sit down, review his or her thinking, and go over all the testing results. If all you get are results mailed to you, you have a right to ask the doctor to give his or her overall analysis. You must have all results explained to you, whether they are normal or abnormal. If there was an x-ray, look at the report. Radiologists always cover themselves. Sometimes they will describe an abnormality, which is more likely normal, but they aren't 100 percent certain. They may add, "I would suggest a further study" if there is suspicion. Similarly, certain blood values may suggest another disease is going on rather than the original one suggested by your doctor.

You are not a physician. So I am not suggesting that you try to diagnose yourself here. However, all studies show that the leading cause of medical malpractice resulting from negligence stems from a wrong initial diagnosis and the failure of the physician to change his or her mind, despite new facts that are contradictory.[3] That means that, once again, the ball is really in your court. Make sure everything is explained to you. Use your logic, your common sense, and even your intuition to determine if what the doctor is telling you makes sense. If it does not, you have a right to a second opinion. Make sure to retain copies of all pertinent testing. You may need this if you talk to another doctor. As I have repeatedly said, doctors make mistakes. Your doctor may have been so busy that he or she subconsciously overlooked an abnormal blood result. The other day, Lisa, a long-standing and close patient, said "Doctor Klein, you said that my tests were normal, but there are two tests that the laboratory noted as abnormal!" Sure enough, my eyes must have glossed over her laboratory slip and failed to register that there were two abnormal liver tests. How unusual, but it proves the point that we, as physicians, make mistakes and sometimes we are not even aware that we do. Fortunately, it turned out to be a laboratory error, but I thanked Lisa and told her she had to continually question all of her doctors, including me. So it is worth repeating that the other lesson I want you to learn (in addition to my drilling in the point again and again about not being afraid to question your doctor) is that you learn from this experience and obtain copies of all tests and results for your own review.

So I subconsciously proved my point. Doctors are human and we all make mistakes. I say this not to let myself and my fellow colleagues off the hook, but to protect you, the patient, from the mistakes that can be made when you believe that your doctor is infallible—or, worse, when your doctor believes that he or she is! The fact is that doctors come to this partnership carrying their own baggage (sometimes an entire monogrammed set of Samsonite), and it is ultimately up to you, the patient, to determine if they are qualified and competent to help you. Are they knowledgeable or caring enough? Will they stay on top of your case? Do they create a safe environment where you feel comfortable sharing your deepest thoughts and concerns? Will they protect you, as the captain of the medical ship, from the often rough seas of the hospital environment?

In this complex mix of patients' needs and fears, as well as those of physicians, there has to be a way for both to unite positively. And that, finally, is the true aim of this chapter: to begin a dialogue that will help you and your doctor create a powerful partnership for achieving optimal health. Your physician must be able to hear you, understand you, and use all of your cues to come up with a fitting and effective diagnosis and a treatment plan. But you, the patient, are not along for a free ride. As it is the physician's role to cure, it is the modern patient's role to be an active participant. You are empowered to protect yourself and always be on the alert for mistakes. But you must be on a quest to know all there is to know about your illness and your options. You are not a passenger, but the copilot, along with your doctor, on this flight toward total well-being. It is not always a smooth ride. There will likely be some choppy weather and turbulence, and you may even get off the flight course at times. But as long as you and your doctor continue to navigate together, you will make the necessary course corrections to keep on track toward your destination, and hopefully, and happily, guide you to that safe landing of true and lasting health.

The National Data Bank and State Professional Licensing Bureau can usually tell you how many malpractice cases your prospective physician has been involved in, although most cases of office malpractice are never made known and therefore do not become part of the statistics. The feeling among most analysts is that many malpractice cases either begin or are limited to your physician's office (this is estimated at 36 percent).[4] That is, the PCP develops a diagnosis and treatment plan, which, if wrong, may lead to the patient winding up in the hospital for a procedure or operation (and the inherent complications) for the wrong reason. Or the patient may undergo some form of malpractice but never know that a mistake was made.

As an example of the latter, a patient may receive the wrong treatment and worsen or may receive a medication that he or she is allergic to, but the doctor has forgotten about the allergy. It is easy to blame the "worsening" on the disease ("Your infection really got worse and there was nothing I could have done. Thank goodness I came up with a better medicine!"). You may have been given antibiotics that would hide a serious underlying infection, making it difficult to diagnose and properly treat. But you survived, even though it took weeks or months to get over the "virus."

A SOFT BELLY AND A HARD HEAD

Recently, my head nurse's 20-year-old daughter developed some lower abdominal pain, which necessitated a local emergency room visit. The girl had fever, abdominal pain, and some tenderness in the lowest point of her abdomen, on the right side. Her abdominal examination showed a soft abdomen (usually not a sign of a serious illness, unless she had taken a narcotic). The on-call surgeon rightly ordered a blood count, blood screen, and a CT scan of the abdomen. The CT scan showed a normal gall bladder, normal organs, and no acute process. The tip of the appendix was not viewable, but there were no signs of any rupture of any organ, including the appendix. The patient's white blood count was low normal at 3,000. But during the twelve hours of her illness, a lymph node enlarged on her neck. That prompted the physician to do a mononucleosis test. When this test also returned normal, the surgeon told the family that *surgery* was necessary as it probably was a diseased appendix that could not be visualized because of some technical problem. In other words, *exploratory* surgery. You know, get under the hood, kick a few tires around, and see if it springs a leak.

Don't get me wrong. Sometimes, after every option has been exhausted and the patient is still suffering, exploratory surgery is a legitimate next step.

But let's look at this a little closer. Was every option explored first? Was this examination truly thorough or was there some other agenda here besides giving the patient the best care possible? All hidden motives aside, there was more to the story that was not being accounted for. For one thing, the patient was in the middle of her menstrual cycle. This significant fact was not sought out by any of the treating physicians. Furthermore, information that was withheld from the family, who now had to make a decision regarding surgery, was that the CT scan showed fluid in the cul-de-sac, an area surrounding the ovaries.

The surgeon should have told the family about this, as it is very suggestive of a ruptured ovarian follicle, common to women, especially during the middle of their menstrual cycle (we call that middle schmertz). The fact that this was withheld from the review process (it was clearly written on the x-ray slip) suggests that the surgeon either did not read that portion or ignored it because it differed from what he had already concluded in his mind. No explanation was given for a normal or low white count, which is usually counter to an acute infectious process, such as appendicitis (low white counts can occur in seriously infected very young children and very old people). The patient was 20 and did not exhibit signs of an overwhelming infection. The final pathology report of the appendix was that it was normal. The swollen lymph gland turned out to be a concomitant mononucleosis infection. And the physicians did not even inform the family that quite often the mono test will be negative for up to two to three weeks. The final diagnosis: The patient actually ruptured an ovarian follicle, the evidence of which was right there on the x-ray.

There were plenty of signs that indicated it was not appendicitis, and plenty of signs that is was, indeed, something else. But once the doctor had made up his mind, a cognitive blind spot occurred that made it difficult for him to see anything else. Either that or he just did not care enough to take the time to make an accurate diagnosis. I am giving him the benefit of the doubt on this one. But when your health or that of a loved one is on the line, you cannot be so generous. You must be the final say. You must become informed, review all the reasoning offered by the physician, go over every lab or x-ray value (normal or not), and get a second opinion, if needed, before making the final decision. The doctors have a lot of other things on their minds—other patients, other problems. You must, therefore, have only one thing on *your* mind—getting the best diagnosis and treatment you possibly can.

Just in case you are not yet convinced of your need to take charge of your medical evaluation when you make an office visit and are not sufficiently fired up so that you never forget it, let me cite a few more examples.

GIVE ME A DOUBLE VISION WITH A TWIST OF LYME

I recently reviewed a medical malpractice case of a young man who developed double vision and was sent to a leading neuro-ophthalmologist for care and treatment. Although the patient had a febrile illness two months previously (in the middle of the summer in Lyme-infested Westchester County), neither the PCP nor the specialist thought to test for this curable disease. They actually did not look for any cause of this acute nerve palsy. The patient went on from one neurological complication to another, ultimately developing Lyme arthritis.

OLD WORLD LOYALTY HAS TO GO

My wife's grandmother, Ruth, developed fevers and swelling around her recently replaced artificial knee following a fall. Her local small town orthopedist guessed, correctly, that she suffered with a knee infection and immediately started her on intravenous antibiotics. The treatment lasted six weeks, which was appropriate. What was not appropriate? You know the answer. It was the fact that the doctor never did any culturing; he believed the infecting organism was due to a particular bacteria and that is what he treated her for. When her fever returned after the six weeks of treatment, his treatment was to repeat the same antibiotic again and again.

Trying to gently encourage an elderly patient to get another opinion is extremely difficult, if not impossible. Ruth lived in this small community for years and was loyal to her physicians. As far as she was concerned, they could do no wrong (if only she had read the previous anecdotes). The family knew things were amiss, but nobody could convince Grandmother. After four months of the same see-saw regimen with no hope in sight, Ruth finally gave in. She was transferred to an orthopedic hospital where all antibiotics were stopped for two weeks. Cultures were then obtained, which revealed the real culprit, which was obviously quite different from that assumed by her community physician. The infection was finally eradicated and Ruth can walk and dance once more. Stubborn loyalty to a physician, who was stubborn himself (as well as unknowledgeable) for not getting his head out of the sand, led to an unnecessary four months of suffering.

JUST A STROKE OF BAD LUCK?

I testified at a malpractice case that involved a middle-age patient who had undergone a prostate biopsy. Three days later he was in his internist's office for his blood pressure check and he informed his physician that he had some chills and a low grade fever. The physician examined the patient's urine with a dip stick test (a stick of chemicals that change colors if there are abnormalities). Sure enough, the indicator for microscopic blood lit up (there is almost always microscopic bleeding after a prostate biopsy), but without a positive indication of white blood cells (the cells that arrive, like the cavalry, to fight infection) and without sending the urine for a culture to prove if there was an infection.

The physician gave the patient an oral antibiotic. Sure enough, the patient felt better; however, when the antibiotic ran out, the fever returned. The physician reordered the antibiotic, not once, but twice more. Each time no urine was taken and no culture was obtained. The physician had made up his mind once, without any proof, that the patient had a urine infection and never took his head out of the sand. The patient really had endocarditis, an infection of the heart valve, which occurred at the time of the original biopsy. The bacteria invaded the patient's valve and stayed there, chewing and chewing away. Only when the oral antibiotic was given did the bacteria take a temporary break. Oral antibiotics are sufficient to cure ordinary urinary infections but do not attain high enough blood levels to cure a heart valve infection. And after two months of this ill-advised treatment based on a lazy diagnosis, the patient was found on the floor of his home, having suffered a major irreversible stroke (a piece of the infection from his diseased valve broke off and clogged a cerebral artery).

An improper diagnosis in a physician's office led to an improper treatment. And the physician never gave a thought to the possibility that there might have been something else wrong.

THE PATIENT BRUSH-OFF

Another case involved a woman who had a simple cyst removed from her finger at her dermatologist's office. She was properly advised of the possible complications (bleeding, infection, recurrence) and home she went. Two days later, she presented to her dermatologist's office with swelling and pain. The physician's assistant, who covered the office when the physician was out or too busy, injected her finger with cortisone (for whatever reason). Over the next two weeks, the finger swelled more and the redness worsened. The dermatologist tried reassuring the woman that it was just some local reaction to surgery. An emergency room physician (where she went after the third week) started her on oral antibiotics and suggested she see her PCP. Two days later, she had an appointment, was told she possibly had a deep infection, and was sent for an orthopedic appointment (rather than having tests done for the deeper infection).

Four days later she was seen by the orthopedist, who did an x-ray, which he read as negative for osteomyelitis (the deeper infection). He continued the oral antibiotics, *which hadn't worked over the past six or seven days*. The patient was now four to five weeks into her infection, and a proper diagnosis and treatment had not yet been arrived at. She went another two weeks before the proper test, an MRI, was done which found the osteomyelitis. The longer the delay there is in the treatment of a disease, the poorer the outcome. This is especially true in the field of infectious diseases. The infection could have spread to this woman's heart or to her brain. The worst that happened—pain, suffering, and deformity—were bad enough. It is interesting that the dermatologist had her sign a piece of paper warning about some of the consequences of the surgery (infection being one of them), but he never thought of that himself in her diagnosis. Perhaps one of the best suggestions one can give a doctor is to read his own paperwork!

WHAT WE'VE GOT HERE IS A FAILURE TO COMMUNICATE

A common form of medical malpractice that occurs in physicians' offices is failure to communicate. Frequently, test results arrive and the office or the physician does not communicate them to the patient in a timely manner.[5] One case I testified at involved a nurse who felt ill and, after her examination by her physician, she asked for a Lyme test. The test proved positive, but the physician never acknowledged the results. In fact, the woman was seen two or three times by her physician over the next few months, complaining of joint pains and ultimately, joint swelling. She subsequently went to a rheumatologist who ordered another Lyme test. This new test was positive for the old Lyme disease and, after checking with the laboratory (he was in the same multispecialty group as the woman's internist), he found the old acutely positive Lyme test of five months earlier. Unfortunately, for the patient, she was to suffer for a few more years before all of her symptoms would dissipate.

As I mentioned earlier with my own patient Lisa, this is a common circumstance. Doctors are busy. Yes, we are usually attentive, however we review thirty or forty sets of test results a day (laboratory, x-ray, electrocardiograms, MRI), and can easily overlook an abnormal result. Adding to this dilemma of worsening good care is the assumption by patients that their tests were normal because their physician did not call to tell them different. It is never a good idea to assume a test is normal just because your doctor did not call. What if the laboratory lost the specimen and, therefore, the doctor never received the results? What if the clerk filed the results away without the doctor reviewing them? What if, as in my case, the doctor saw the results but because of inattentiveness, the results did not "register"? Patients must be empowered to be their own advocates. Did you ask the doctor for the results? Did you get a copy and see the results for yourself?

In this case of Lyme disease (it is Lyme and not Lymes), the symptoms, as in many other diseases, can initially disappear as the body's first line of defense stalls the bacterial invasion. Weeks to months later, the secondary and tertiary complications set in and that is when trouble will rear its ugly head.

DOCTORS' DIRTY LITTLE SECRETS

A recent in-depth interview with 53 family physicians revealed that 47 percent of the doctors (nearly half) had a case where a patient died due to physician error.[6] Only four of these cases led to a malpractice suit. That is, approximately 10 percent were sued. An editorial article in the *New York*

Times summarized a study reported in the *Archives of Internal Medicine*. In it, 2,600 doctors in the United States and Canada confirmed that they were less likely to admit a serious mistake if they thought they could get away with it. Ninety-eight percent of the doctors endorsed the need to disclose any serious error to the patient, but only half of the doctors would actually use the word "error." It was found that many of the doctors would only admit to a mistake if the mistake became overtly obvious (a sponge left in after surgery, requiring another operation). If the error was too subtle for most patients to recognize, most of the doctors would not admit an error had been made. The researchers suggested that placing limits on malpractice claims would not have any impact on what doctors admitted.[7]

A colleague of mine admitted to destroying a cardiogram that he misread when finding out that the patient went to the hospital that same night and died of a heart attack. The cardiogram had been grossly abnormal and the physician did not really study it well. Had he seen the abnormal changes, the patient would not have died. The tainted evidence was easily destroyed without a trace of culpability. Usually most office malpractice errors will not have a bad outcome, and most cases will never be known to the patients. If the error causes the patient to be admitted to the hospital, then the outcomes seriously worsen.[8]

One case of such doctor denial that I sat through was that of Mrs. Mercer. She had gone upstate New York to visit friends in a town called Hyde Park, about a two-hour car ride north of New York City. Two weeks later, she sought medical advice when she developed a flulike illness (fever, malaise, and chills). When she was examined, she pointed out a rash behind her right knee. Her physician told her it was a virus and that she should take aspirin and fluids. Three days later, she called complaining of no improvement. Her physician was off but, for some unknown reason, she did not speak to either of his partners. Two days later, she was feeling weak and had a mild fever. She now had many large blotches of redness (a rash) over her body and was seen again by her physician. She again told him of her trip to upstate New York (where Lyme disease is prevalent). "No, this is not the classic rash of Lyme disease but I don't know what it is," the doctor said. He made an appointment with a dermatologist for two days later. The visit was too late. She awoke the next day with Bell's palsy (the drooping of one side of her face). After the dermatologist diagnosed correctly that she *did* have Lyme disease, she was sent to a well-known neurologist. This prominent physician proceeded to put her on oral antibiotics instead of intravenous antibiotics, which is the recommended treatment for neurological complications (if the doctor had just used Google, he would have discovered that! Forget the fact that, as a neurologist, he should have known!). This is another reason why you, the patient, should use that ubiquitous search tool Google. (Of course, not everything you find will be true or accurate, but the corroboration of multiple sources of information will certainly make you a more informed patient.) Remember Sy Simms's motto.

We know the patient saw her physician in a timely manner, and we know that the patient came down with oftentimes reversible paralysis of half of her face. But you must also know that the physician will, to his last breath, deny any culpability. He will hire the fanciest lawyer and pay thousands of dollars in fees to argue that it was not his fault. His reasoning will be that the rash was not classic—many people travel upstate and do not come back with Lyme disease. Forget the fact that New York, and most of the surrounding states, are well known for Lyme disease. Forget the fact that the area north of New York City is the *epicenter* for this disease in the northeast. A lesson I teach my medical students is that anyone who has the summer flu with fever has Lyme disease until proven otherwise. And Lyme can present as any type of rash, not just as the classic bull's-eye that one reads about. Any practicing physician in that area worth his or her license should know and consider that. I like to remind my colleagues about my alma mater, the University of Rome. Near the ancient campus compound, there is a large and impressive building to the immediate right. It bears the name The Institute for Syphilis and Dermatology. Interesting combination, no? What could the link possibly be between dermatology and history's most famous venereal disease? The pairing cracks open the door to any number of jokes, but the fact that it is carved above the entrance to a departmental building at one of the oldest institutions of higher learning in the Western world leaves many scratching their heads.

Before the antibiotic era, when syphilis was rampant, the rashes caused by this disease were plentiful and diverse beyond the initial skin ulcerations in the genital area. Therefore, the presentation of any rash or skin lesion always contained syphilis as part of the differential diagnosis: it was so prevalent that it deserved equal billing with dermatology. To get to the point, both syphilis and Lyme are caused by a similar bacteria, a spirochete, which can show itself by many different types of rashes.

But more important, why did the doctor have to deny that he obviously made a mistake (especially when it is *so* obvious)? Is it the unwillingness to believe that he is capable of making a mistake or not wanting to have an "insurance" record of mistakes? Either way, it is a flaw in the system that consistently leads to errors and omissions, which leads to a lack of understanding, and, ultimately, the wisdom that could prevent the problems in the future. This, of course, means more people get sicker and even die—unnecessarily.

The fact is, Mrs. Mercer got sick and developed complications on his watch. He did not cause the disease, but he failed to recognize it. He made a mistake in diagnosis. That happens all the time and doctors must have the courage to admit it instead of fearing that they won't be covered by malpractice insurance. Furthermore, insurance companies should allow doctors to admit errors. As it now stands, if a doctor admits an error, his malpractice insurer can drop the case and not be responsible for any damages. It states this on the malpractice contracts we sign.[9] Many malpractice educational programs, participation in which is encouraged by these malpractice insurance companies, are now suggesting that perhaps we could tell patients if we make a mistake. But the insurance companies still make you sign the waiver that you cannot. The insurer would have difficulty defending a case when the doctor admitted responsibility. Even the greatest of lawyers have difficulty defending against a confession. Nobody should deny compensation to an injured patient if the injury was caused by malpractice. But that is the way our present system works. Do not admit to wrong doing. There may be some lawyer who can prove it was not your fault that you cut off the wrong foot. If we are not allowed to admit guilt, the system will remain broken and will eventually collapse under the weight of its own burden.

Most cases I see are just like that. The doctor sees the patient, makes the wrong diagnosis, the patient develops a complication from the mistaken diagnosis, the patient goes to court, and the insurance carrier denies his or her part. Earlier, I mentioned the case of a woman who developed osteomyelitis after her dermatologist operated on her finger. The patient originally had a cyst. The dermatologist performed three procedures on the cyst and the patient went on to develop a deep-seated bone infection. In court, the physician denied he did anything to cause the infection. I sat there in disbelief. It is bad enough that a patient is harmed by a mistake. But to watch the person you trusted with your health sit there and downright lie . . . it is a form of violation that ranks up there. Ultimately, the doctor's defense attorney sufficiently twisted things out of context, confused the jury with bells and whistles, and the patient lost her case because the doctor had a better, perhaps higher-paid, lawyer.

Doctors not only lie to you, the patient, they lie to other physicians, thinking that they can get away with it. A patient of mine was having a benign growth removed from her ovary and underwent gynecological surgery at a nearby hospital (at which I do not attend and therefore did not know the gynecologist). One week later, the patient's mom called me in hysteria that her daughter had been in the intensive care unit of the hospital, near death, for the past five days. I got the doctor's name and called him. "Oh," he said, "the surgery went fine but two days later she had a diverticula (out pouching of the large intestine) perforate and she developed acute peritonitis, which we didn't pick up for a day or so. So they had to go in a second time to remove the diseased intestine." Now that is the kind of stuff that is outlandish. What are the odds of somebody having a ruptured intestine a day or so after surgery? Seems that something was being hidden and you can guess along with me that perhaps the gynecologist did something wrong. So I called the pathology department at that hospital and explained that I was her physician. He kindly sent me the pathology report on the "diseased" intestine, which had a laceration through it and not a ruptured diverticula. Thankfully the hospital has to examine and save the surgical specimen. The gynecologist perforated the intestine while doing his surgery and tried to absolve himself from blame. It will be interesting if he stated the ruptured diverticula as the cause in his medical records. This would be contrary to the pathology report, and would have made for a nice medical malpractice case.

The majority of office medical injuries, however, do not directly lead to death and maiming, because there are very few life-threatening invasive procedures done in private offices. Bad outcomes of "missed" diagnoses in offices usually end up in the hospital. Here, statistics show, for every six medical injuries occurring, one patient will die.[10]

However, the overall incidence of medical malpractice in offices is much higher than estimated.[11] Unlike hospital records, private office records are more easily altered. Laboratory and x-ray records can be easily destroyed. Hospital records are usually unalterable and malpractice more easily traceable. I testified at a case two years ago where a state agency was asked to look into the unexpected death of an inpatient. The state copied the records for review, unbeknownst to the treating physician. Usually, if a patient, lawyer, or the patient's family requests copies of hospital records, the treating physician is notified as a courtesy. In this instance, no one was notified when the state agency copied the records. When the case went to court, the doctor's hospital records were different from the original records. This was picked up by the state's lawyer, who noted the "doctored" physician's progress notes, obviously rewritten to hide any misconduct. It usually is quite difficult to change hospital records, and although the doctor almost got away with it, justice prevailed and he lost his medical license.

Most physicians mean well and are not evil. The negative climate of malpractice, as it is seen today, can cause physicians to lie or cheat. The hope is that we can change everyone's outlook and be able to acknowledge that we, physicians, are not perfect and admit our errors. Obviously, the goal is not to have a country full of error-admitting physicians. The aim is to lower the error rate. Not only will this change in attitude strengthen the bond between patient and physician, but it will also help prevent future errors and accidents. The bottom line is that you, the patient, deserve an explicit acknowledgment of error, information about why it happened and, at the very least, an apology.

Changes in medical education and encouraging disclosure would help. Furthermore, computerized systems to detect errors are needed that would otherwise remain unnoticed and help lead to eradication of these errors. There has to be a national registry where all of these errors and mistakes are computerized and analyzed. Physicians and hospitals would report errors without fear of being punished. Nor would the reporting physicians' or hospitals' names be made known to the public. The errors should be publicized so that the consumers can also know what to look for. The results would be for teaching and learning how to avoid the same pitfalls, thereby cutting down on the amount of errors.

I have a patient who is a surgeon and his operating infection rate was qua-druple all other surgeons at his hospital for the same procedures. This was a fact that was not known by the public at large nor by most of his referring physicians. The hospital had not approached him or tried to evaluate his technique. This makes no sense. When he informed me recently of this high rate of infection, which had been going on for years, I sent him for skin cul-tures. Sure enough, the surgeon had many unusual bacteria growing on his skin. The problem was identified and the cure was in showering twice daily with hexachlorophene soap. His infection rate is now the same as his peers.

Of a list of surgical adverse reactions, infection is one of the highest ac-ceptable complications. This will be dealt with in Chapter 13. However, if theoretically the average surgical risk were 5 percent for a gallbladder re-moval (a number I just made up) and a particular surgeon has an infection rate of 30 percent, that is not acceptable. That is malpractice. Even today some juries in malpractice cases are not allowed to know what the surgeon's infection rate is, compared to acceptable standards, or his or her prior malpractice history. Surgical infections are usually not caused by multiple rare bacterial colonizations on the skin (such as the general surgeon I men-tioned). First and foremost, in 99 percent of clean surgeries, the infection is put into the surgical site at the time of surgery. Once the wound is closed, you can sprinkle bacteria over the wound and they would not be able to get into this sealed environment. A gunshot wound to the abdomen is dirty surgery as compared to a clean, elective gallbladder removal. At the time of surgery, the introduced bacteria arise from the failure of properly sterilizing the environment. There is a break in sterile technique, and it is usually the patient's own bacteria, which was not properly cleansed, that is introduced into the wound. That is, the patient's skin was not cleansed properly. To further complicate things, if a patient has an infection on some other part of his or her body, there will be a good chance that the same bacteria will wind up in the wound. Other than not cleansing the patient adequately, bacteria can come from many other sources, such as the surgeon, surgical assistant, infected instruments, and so forth. I would take it with a grain of salt if a surgeon tells you that the bacteria got into the wound two days later because you scratched yourself or because the wound got wet. Remember, as resi-dents in training we used to kid about how surgeons never ever believe that they are the cause of a surgical wound infection. Even though they make you sign a piece of paper stating it isn't so, that could be one of the complications. They or someone in the operating room are usually the cause.

I had not spoken with my friend Hal in years and he called recently to wish me a happy New Year. Then he proceeded to tell me about his terrible back surgery and its many complications. He told me that he had lumbar surgery for a herniated disc. Two weeks later, he was back in the hospital with a terrible wound infection, causing him ultimately to come down with meningitis. The infection had spread into his spinal cord, because it was in the nearby disc space. His surgeon told him later that it, the infection, probably was because he had a shower two weeks after surgery. How dis-ingenuous of the surgeon. It is true, no one wants to admit responsibility and get sued. But the surgeon knows, just as I know, that the infection is almost always put in the wound at the time of the original surgery.

The American Society of Anesthesiology did an in-depth analysis of the most common types of errors performed by sending questionnaires to their members. By statistically studying surveys of thousands of anesthesiologists, a set of guidelines was developed. The result: the nationwide error rate for this group was decreased by 50 percent.[12] In other words, bringing awareness to this problem and holding people accountable help to eradicate the problem. And that saves lives.

I further propose that patients should have access to a physicians "report card" (not from information supplied to the National Registry). The report would consist of the amount of malpractice claims and losses and the physician's infection or complication rates. Poor grades would require extra training. In the meantime, you can take steps to create a report card of your own. While you may not be able to obtain all the necessary information to create a complete picture of your doctor's grade level, with a few phone calls, some Googling, and a bit of sleuthing you can begin to get a much more accurate sense of who you are dealing with. And as more patients take this kind of control, more doctors will stop taking their positions for granted and take their practice to the next level.

Remember, statistics show that 5 percent of our practicing physicians are responsible for 50 percent of malpractice payments.[13] Until now nothing has been done to this 5 percent. Should they be identified and legally forced to be retrained? Should they have to practice under the guidance of another physician? Nothing has been done to improve their abilities. These physicians are still practicing, without any sanctions by their respective state licensing authorities. I am presently preparing to testify against a physician who had lost her license five years ago, for a period of three years. Her offense was treating dozens of patients for a disease they did not have, not diagnosing them with the proper disease, and using all sorts of witchcraft and bogus injections that would not work on any infection. She told all of these adult patients that they were suffering with chronic mononucleosis. Now that is a diagnosis that can be proved by doing the appropriate testing. All of the tests that this physician performed were negative for chronic mononucleosis (that is they failed to prove the existence of this infection). She gave these patients injections of gamma globulin and vitamin B_{12}, as well as a host of other medications. She treated them all for years and years, carrying this diagnosis, when in actuality they suffered from serious, life-threatening diseases (one patient had leukemia). Yes, the physician deserved to lose her license, but she came back. You cannot teach a leopard to lose its spots, and similarly this physician went on to practice the same medicine as before. She started treating patients again for chronic mononucleosis, despite the lack of laboratory confirmation. Unfortunately, there was one woman who complained of back pain, which progressed and progressed. Of course this physician told her that it was because of the chronic mononucleosis. To get to the point, at the end of eight months of suffering, the patient wound up in an emergency room, where an x-ray, yes an x-ray, was finally taken which showed that the patient had bone cancer that had spread from her lungs. The family of this now deceased woman is suing the physician, who never should have been allowed back into medicine or, at the very least, should have been closely monitored by the state authorities. I have to reiterate, mistakes can be and are made by any physician.

Unlike years ago when the local doctor was godlike, today we as patients must question everyone and everything. We know that millions of errors occur yearly. We must do whatever we can to make sure we are not the victims of one. As more patients begin taking an active role in their health care, asking questions, pointing out problems when they suspect medical malpractice, and raising their voices to their political representatives, the momentum this will create will lead to real change.

As a final note on the subject of system changes, to better aid caring for patients, physicians should initiate online record keeping. This would allow records to be available, online, in real time. These records would be set up to prevent deletion, although new information could be subsequently added, and the records could be viewed by health care workers anywhere in the world (obviously, with proper permission). Patients' electrocardiograms, laboratory data, x-rays, and other information would be available for review in real time if a patient were ill at a different location. Think of the benefits of such a system. Two patients within the past two months had symptoms suggestive of heart disease. Each had separately had a stress test at their previous cardiologist's offices, which I had been unaware of. Remember, just like Michael, who informs me if he went to another physician and if a test had been done, he would produce a copy of the test and the results; you must do the same. The cardiologists failed to send me the results and the patients never told me, their primary care physician, that tests had been done. Getting copies of these tests is important for the PCP so he or she can review them as well. In these two cases, the patients were told that their tests were normal, but they were not. They were both walking around with cardiac time bombs, thinking themselves healthy, when the truth lay in reviewing of the tests. Both went on to cardiac catheterization and both are now healthy. I will discuss this in detail in Chapter 7. Until online record keeping exists, one thing you can do is at least keep copies of all pertinent test results and diagnoses. Perhaps it could be kept on a small thumbnail drive that you could travel with, in case of medical emergencies. Or perhaps it could be put on a personal, password-protected Web page. The point is, there are options. Despite the flaws in the system, there are many things you can do to prevent becoming a victim of it. If you get nothing else from this, my hope is that you accept that premise and begin to operate from it in your future interactions with the medical industry.

Most motor vehicle accidents occur within a few miles of one's home or physician. That's one argument for *not* going to your doctor. But let me give you a few more facts that will better prepare you for that medical experience that might be around the corner.

IMPORTANCE OF UPDATING YOUR ADDRESS

Alice was a baggage handler for a major airline and sought relief from a flulike illness in June 1999. Her physician smartly drew a blood specimen for Lyme disease. The following week, the test was reported as positive but for some reason did not arrive on the proper physician's desk for another two weeks. The nurse placed phone calls, but the line was disconnected and they could not get in touch with the patient. It turns out Alice had moved months before and had never given her new forwarding telephone number or mailing address.

The physician, in her examination before trial (EBT), claimed that a letter was sent to Alice but was returned because of a lack of a forwarding address. The only proof of this was a copy of the letter and not its envelope. As is usually the case, acute Lyme disease is self-limiting and Alice seemingly got over her illness naturally. She therefore did not bother calling for any blood test results. Four or five months later, however, Alice started experiencing severe arthritic complaints with major swelling and disability of her left knee. When she went back to her physician, she discovered she had had Lyme all that time, which had gone untreated.

She was now experiencing the complications of secondary Lyme disease, Lyme arthritis. The physician prescribed oral antibiotics for one month. During this period, Alice's condition worsened. She lost weight as well as strength. Her mental cognitive functions diminished and, needless to say, her arthritis worsened. At the end of the month, Alice went on disability because she could not lift bags anymore. She was sent to an infectious disease expert and finally started on the proper course of intravenous antibiotics. Acute Lyme is successfully treated with oral antibiotics. However, the sequelae (complications such as arthritis) should be treated intravenously. After all of these examples, you will unlikely forget that treatment.

Alice sued her physician because of a delay in notifying her, thereby allowing her disease to worsen. There was a three-week period where the doctor should have received the blood results. That wasn't the doctor's fault, but certainly not within the standards expected in our community. Telephoning the patient was an attempt, but sending a registered letter would have been more in keeping with proper notification, as there usually is a forwarding address. At least a registered letter would have given proof that an attempt was made.

I testified in this case two years after the malpractice suit was instituted. Reviewing her chart two years later, I found her work number at the airline listed under the place of business section. Two years after she had stopped working, the airline number (her place of business) had not been changed. Alice could have been notified because she was first seen while she was fully employed. Furthermore, the office had kept a copy of her copay check from the original office visit when her blood was taken for Lyme as part of her record. The check had her new address on it. My testimony dealt with what would have happened to Alice if there had not been a delay in treatment (in this case there was by a delay in notification). Obviously, by treating her in a timely and proper fashion, she would have been cured. Unfortunately, Alice was treated from the start with the wrong modality: she should have received intravenous and not oral antibiotics.

But the real issue here is not the mistake the doctor's office made *after* the delay in communication; the lesson here is that all of this could have been avoided by Alice. Had she called for her blood results, rather than just assuming that, since she was feeling better, the doctor would have called her if something was wrong, her years of suffering and heartache would have been avoided entirely. Don't get me wrong, I'm not siding with the doctor. In fact, I found in favor of the plaintiff. What I am saying is that the ball really was in her court. And that is the message I want you to take away. Yes, the doctor made mistakes. So what! That will offer you little comfort when you or a loved one suffers irreversible complications from an event that you could have prevented by making a simple phone call for test results or making sure the doctor had your correct contact information.

PICKING THE RIGHT DOCTOR

After choosing the right insurance company, choosing the right doctor is the most important step in protecting yourself from medical injury. Doctors are ranked in their medical school class. That ranking, however, may not hold true as to the quality of physician one ultimately becomes. For example, they were not graded on empathy, caring, and inquisitiveness. Neither were they graded on fact finding or solving the ultimate puzzle. Once fully matured, physicians attain a new ranking, which has nothing to do with prior grades. Nevertheless, most medical mistakes are made by a handful of less-than-excellent doctors. Statistically speaking, 5 percent of practicing physicians cause 50 percent of all malpractice hospital deaths. Again, yes, mistakes can be, and are, made by most physicians at some time in their careers.

There are many other factors that lead to bad physicians (or bad practice habits):

- Being overworked
- Being unhappy at home
- Personal and mental problems (which worsen as one ages)
- Political and peer pressure from hospitals
- Insurance companies (which compare the amounts of testing and use of specialists to similar physicians in the area, or the amount of CT scans or other test ordered)

Referrals from neighbors and patients may tell you how concerned and sincere your next physician is; however, they won't really tell you about his or her medical abilities. Only other physicians have knowledge and insights into the quality of care practiced by other physicians. So if you want to know who is a good doctor, ask another doctor whom they would see if they were sick.

My son Brian was away at college when he called one evening to say he had been ill for the past day and got worse that afternoon, losing his appetite for those delicious homemade cookies he received. Now that is an admission of being ill! He had gone to the student health center, but it was now closed at 5 P.M. His next stop was the local emergency room. And by the time I flew to his college in Syracuse, New York, he was already under anesthesia and under the knife, having his diseased appendix removed by the on-call surgeon.

Who knew how good that surgeon was? Fortunately, Brian did just fine. But the experience taught me a strong lesson. From then on, any time a family member was going to be gone for an extended period (school, work), I called the local hospitals and spoke with the chiefs of service. I obtained names of internists and surgeons who they thought were good. I then requested that my children make "well" appointments with the internists, becoming an official patient. This way, a good physician, or his or her covering staff, would be in charge in case of an emergency. This is a proactive practice I strongly encourage you to adopt.

Physician recommendation is very important. Hospital affiliation is also up there and will be discussed later. Great physicians still make medical errors and we must still, therefore, be vigilant and active participants in our own care. The likelihood, however, is usually a lot less for a doctor with a proven track record of excellent care. Bottom line, it is a numbers game. And doing this kind of due diligence *before* there is a medical crisis will increase your odds of receiving better care.

HOW NOT TO PICK THE RIGHT DOCTOR

I recently saw a gentleman as an infectious disease consultation for swelling and cellulites of his face. Unfortunately, Pat had been in and out of the hospital for short bouts of intravenous antibiotics (two days each, separated by two days). He had no improvement in his infection. The point is not to stress the importance of continuous intravenous therapy, rather than an intravenous treatment here and there. The real problem was when I called the infectious disease specialist caring for him. It turned out he was someone I had known thirty years ago and had not seen since. "Oh, that guy is a real pain," the specialist told me. "He Googles everything and asks too many questions." Let me make no bones about it—that physician turned out to be a real jerk. He represented the antithesis of this book. He was not open or willing to participate in collaboration with his patient. As a result, no one made the proper diagnosis. Perhaps this lack of success, and the resulting bruise to his ego, compelled this doctor to devalue this patient's input. After all, it was either that or admit that he was in error. Or maybe it was the fact that the patient left him for another doctor—me. Sadly, this type of arrogance even goes so far as to blame the patient for not getting better. "I never had a patient that didn't get better with what you have," the doctor might say, in an effort to alleviate all responsibility from himself. "You must have done something," he will add. "Did you wet it? Did you dry it?"

QUESTION, QUESTION, QUESTION!

Then there was the doctor who admitted his patient into the hospital suffering from anemia and having chest pains. Acutely anemic patients can exhibit cardiac symptoms (especially if elderly), as the lowered hemoglobin (red blood cells) carries less oxygen than is needed. People with underlying heart disease already have a "strain" on their oxygen supply because of blockage of the flow of blood to the coronary arteries (which feed the heart muscle). Rather than doing a rectal examination to see whether the anemia was due to gastrointestinal bleeding (which is a major cause of acute anemia) and which is standard protocol, the physician ordered stool cards to be sent to the laboratory. This test takes a few days whereas the rectal test will give immediate results. After three days, the cardiologist deemed that there was no acute cardiac disease or event and scheduled the patient for an outpatient stress test. He recommended discharge.Just prior to the patient going home, the laboratory called the admitting physician and informed him that the stool cards were positive (that there was blood present in the stool). This should have been a warning to the doctor but he decided to ignore this important piece of information and discharged the patient, instructing him to see a gastroenterologist later that week. The patient should have been kept in the hospital for an immediate evaluation, which is the normal standard of care. Two days later, the patient was readmitted as an emergency, suffering from a massive gastrointestinal bleed and peritonitis, caused by a penetrating gastric ulcer (which ate its way through the stomach wall). The patient was in shock and required multiple surgeries because of the complications of this unnecessary disaster. Gastric ulcers are known to cause chest pain, and this was the original symptom the patient presented at the emergency room.

Many of us are still fearful of doctors and what they say to us. Sometimes they say something that sounds ominous, something we do not understand, and we leave their office preoccupied with their last statement. Did he mean that I have cancer? Did she say I was getting worse? We then spend the weekend ruminating over that last phrase. We don't sleep, we go to work thinking it may be our last day. Why didn't I ask him what he meant? On and on the mental suffering goes.

Well that was yesterday's tradition! From today forth, you will not leave a doctor's office until you fully understand everything that has been said. I would rather your physician get frazzled a little than have you spend one sleepless night, worried about something that could be totally innocuous. I know I have said this before, but you need to ask as many questions as possible. Not only will it help you understand what it is you may or may not have, it also puts your physician on notice that he or she really has to think out loud about the diagnosis. Mention diseases that you are concerned about. It is possible that the physician did not think about them. Perhaps he or she had and these diseases are not even near what you have. Fine. At least you can relax, knowing that these are eliminated. Just remember that the most common cause of medical malpractice is the wrong diagnosis. One only arrives at the right diagnosis if one thinks about it. If your doctor isn't thinking for him- or herself, ask questions until he or she starts.

Study after study shows that you are not alone when it comes to asking questions or telling the doctor that you did not understand what he said. Patients are either embarrassed (after all, the physician is wearing the white coat and is the knowledgeable one) or just not up to knowing medical terminology.[14] Medical terms are confusing, and because most people do not understand or ask for clarification, they are more apt to have poorer care or more complications. Studies further show that death rates among those with limited health literacy are twice as high as those who are literate. Doctors often fail to speak laymen English and, as a consequence, many people (educated or not, rich or poor) will suffer for not speaking up. Insist that your doctor speak plainly. You want to hear: "You don't have HIV," rather than "Your HIV test was negative." What does that mean to the average person? You want to hear: "Do you have pain in your chest when you take a deep breath?" rather than "Do you have pleuritic pain?" To the average person, they might as well be speaking in tongues.[15]

A physician once told me: "One day I had to be the bearer of bad news when I told a wife that her husband had died of a massive myocardial infarct."

Not more than five minutes later, I heard her report to the rest of the family that he had died of a "massive internal fart." Now that may make some people laugh, but I can assure you, it was—and is—no laughing matter.

When I give complicated instructions to my patients (to me that is the equivalent of two or more changes in their prescriptions, or getting a certain test before doing something else), I ask them to repeat to me what it is that I want them to do. Furthermore, I then write out everything on a piece of paper. If your doctor does not have you write things down, then you need to remember to do it for yourself. Additionally, if you are to discuss anything of importance with your physician, make sure you have your clothes on and are in his or her consultation room. This stuff is hard enough to understand fully clothed, you do not need the additional distraction of asking questions half naked! Also, being half dressed puts you on less than an equal par with your physician. If the physician insists that you complete your questions while still undressed, insist that he or she take off his or her clothes too!

Bring paper and pen to your appointment. Even better, bring a spouse or close friend with paper and pen. The best of all is to tape the conversation. This way you can play it again and again, to your spouse or to another physician when you go for a second opinion. Before you leave from this parting consultation, ask yourself: What questions can and should I come up with, rather than the doctor asking "Do you have any questions?" And one more word about second opinions: I love them. Patients have often told me that their prior physicians have blustered or got upset if they questioned their doctor's authority. Unfortunately, there are many immature or insecure physicians who go ballistic if you suggest getting a second opinion. Oftentimes in life bluster is a mechanism for hiding ignorance of the facts. Think about changing your doctor, because that behavior is unacceptable. I encourage second opinions because (a) it is nice if I discover I am right, and (b) it is even better to hear I am wrong *before* the patient suffers. There is an old medical adage that the farther away and more expensive, the better the second opinion. This refers to sending your patient to a major research and teaching center.

This is your health and your life and you must be an active participant. Question. Question. Question. Is the procedure ordered necessary? Are you allergic to the medicine? Will you be allergic to the dye used in the x-ray or scan? I will wager that if you ask your doctor if the medicine that he just prescribed for you (for your sore throat, or congestion, or whatever) was absolutely necessary the answer 50 percent of the time would be no! That is just a guess on my part, but imagine that 50 percent of the time you would probably be putting yourself at risk for a medicine that really is not necessary. Think of how many times you were given an antibiotic for the common cold. They do not work for a virus. Furthermore, according to a *USA Today* article, one of seven commonly used drugs are taken for off-label uses lacking any scientific support.[16] If you had a head cold and suffered with prostate inflammation, cold remedies would cause you to have difficulty urinating. Many people will stay up all night because of the ingredients in cold medicines. But the real concern is that we really do not need half of what our doctors give us. It is as if patients really want something to take for their effort in going to their doctor. The doctor is only obliging. Just try asking.

Contact your state and federal legislators and ask them to fight for a physician's report card as well as a National Registry. Ask them to fight for unalterable electronic records. And ask them to help save our lives as well as theirs. Injuries and deaths are preventable.

PRESCRIPTION

- Bring a list of all of your complaints on your next doctor's visit. Include on this list all names of the medications (prescription, over the counter, and herbal remedies) that you are taking. Another physician may have added or subtracted something that your doctor does not know about.
- Make sure your physician answers each question/problem satisfactorily.
- Look at every laboratory slip, review every positive result with your physician.
- Make sure your name is on each tube of blood removed from you and on your requisition form. (In the next few chapters, you will see that improper labeling is responsible for many injuries to patients.) I asked my nursing staff if they would be insulted or imposed upon if patients requested their double checking. They assured me that they would not mind.
- Make sure your name is on the laboratory or pathology reports when they return.

- Keep copies of every test obtained and the subsequent results.
- Make sure you have your doctor's full attention. Do not ask an important question when he or she is finishing with you and is halfway out the room.
- If possible, get copies of your office notes.
- If you are waiting a long time for your doctor, locked up in an examination room, it is okay to open the door. Perhaps they did forget about you. However, if you stand outside the doorway, with your arms folded in an angry stance, you will get nothing but negative points with the doctor and staff.
- Ask for second opinions.
- Ask for over reads on x-rays done in your physician's office.
- If you feel *any* uneasiness about answers, or if you feel that the doctor is holding back or hiding something, get another opinion.
- Ask if the medicine you are being prescribed is absolutely necessary.

4

DOES YOUR KID REALLY NEED THAT SHOT? PROTECTING YOUR CHILDREN IN THE SYSTEM

Every child comes with a message that God is not yet discouraged of man.

—Rabindranath Tagore[1]

This chapter will discuss the all-important topic of how to handle your children's health care, from the moment they come home to the day they leave (unless they are one of those kids who never leave, in which case this chapter isn't going to help you!). It will walk the reader through the process of how to choose the right pediatrician or family doctor, how to deal with all the dos and don'ts of early care from two weeks on, how to talk about what to look for and how to be your child's best advocate during well visits and sick visits, and address the concerns and controversies around whether or not parents should have their kids immunized completely. I will discuss the use, and potential overuse, of antibiotics on kids, and the long-term consequences on their health, and how to deal with a diagnosis or treatment that you do not feel is right, without being intimidated by the doctor.

The chapter will then break down the most common health concerns or scary symptoms that kids have, when to take them to the doctor, when to keep them home, and how to treat them if you do. It will also touch on the important subject of attention deficit hyperactivity disorder (ADHD) and the epidemic of methylphenidate (Ritalin) and similar drugs. More information, however, on this topic will be contained in Chapter 11. It would be impossible to cover every childhood ailment in this book, and certainly there are everyday health issues that all parents have to deal with, and more extraordinary issues that some parents have to deal with. In all cases, you should view yourself as your child's advocate. He or she cannot ask informed questions or request a second opinion or to see a test result. As your child's only real advocate, it is advisable to ask questions, to keep good notes, and to get second opinions when you feel they are warranted.

Picking a pediatrician is similar to choosing any physician. Having a child late in my life, I asked my fellow younger colleagues whom they would use. Now we have been using our present pediatrician for the past three years. Recently, I had to take Matthew for a checkup and all went well until I was ready to leave the office, when the secretary asked "How much is your co-pay?" That was the first time that question was ever asked of me (we older physicians were brought up with the old world rule of never charging your fellow physician). Psychiatrists say they must charge because of whatever transference, or nontransference, goes on. What was more irksome was that the pediatrician was standing just a few feet away and obviously could hear the conversation. I stammered, "I really have no idea, but please send a bill." Ouch number one. On one occasion my wife said that Matthew wasn't acting right all morning, so she took his temperature, which was 103 degrees. "Well dear," I said, "kids get high fevers all of the time." But to ease her mind I placed a call to the covering physician's answering service. Well mothers' instincts being what they are (and my wife is no exception), Caryn decided to take Matthew to the emergency room rather than wait. Then the covering physician returned my call and said, "Well, kids get high fevers all of the time." Matthew was greeted in the emergency room by needles and his white blood count was an astounding 38,000. That was very, very high. He immediately had blood cultures taken and was started on intravenous antibiotics. He was subsequently discharged and told to follow-up with his regular pediatrician in two days. The pediatrician was also amazed at the very high white count and asked his two partners if they ever saw such a response. When my wife came home, I asked what Matthew's repeat count was and she said that they didn't do one. Ouch number two. When you start getting negative vibes, perhaps it is time to change before real trouble starts.

Pediatricians' offices have the same pitfalls as do adults' physicians' offices (the exception being that kids cannot verbalize their symptoms).

Updated geographics have to be maintained. Parent office demeanor has to be sparkling, and attention to receiving the proper shots and labeling of specimens have to be the same as in adults' physicians' offices.

A few rules to follow as you head into parenthood are:

1. Choose a board-certified obstetrician to deliver your baby and follow his or her advice for prenatal care.
2. If possible, use a hospital with a neonatal intensive care unit that is staffed by board-certified neonatologists, in the rare event that your baby runs into any difficulty.
3. Many hospitals utilize only general pediatricians to care for their newborns but have usually made arrangements to transfer high-risk infants to regional, tertiary care centers if a baby has a problem. If your baby is born by Cesarean section (30 percent of deliveries in the United States), make sure that a pediatrician will be present at the birth to provide any special care if needed.[2] Therefore, choosing the right hospital for your delivery requires research and due diligence.
4. Interview your pediatrician before you use his or her services. Your insurance carrier may or may not pay for this consultation, but then you pay for it anyway. Is he or she certified by and does he or she follow the guidelines set forth by the American Academy of Pediatrics, regarding child care? Does the doctor's personality seem to jive with yours?
5. Try to breast feed: it is healthier because it provides all of the nutrition required during the first six months, it affords a certain degree of protection against illness, it may reduce illness, and it is less expensive than formula.
6. Take folic acid as prescribed by your doctor when trying to conceive, it reduces the incidence of spinal cord defects in the newborn.
7. Vitamins A, C, and D are usually prescribed for breast-fed babies for the first three months of life.

The general rule is that babies are seen in the newborn nursery on a daily basis and for routine well baby care a few days after birth in the doctor's office and then at increasing intervals (i.e., one, three, six, nine, and twelve months during the first year). You get a break during the second year, even the pediatrician does not want to see a child during the terrible two's! Seriously, you get a break and the child is usually seen at 15, 18, and 24 months old.

Exceptions occur if there is an ongoing problem or the doctor is concerned about a questionable abnormal finding he or she wishes to recheck. How many years your child remains with a pediatrician varies. Most make the transition to an internist in their teens. Occasionally, some patients have to be nudged out of the practice in their twenties. "But doctor, I have become so used to you!"

The subspecialty of neonatology (care and treatment of newborn babies) has progressed rapidly during the past forty years. Whereas a very low birth weight previously would spell almost a certain demise for the infant years ago, many weighing as little as two pounds or lower are being saved. Progress can be attributed to many factors including the establishment of regional neonatal intensive care centers, the training of neonatologists, improved technology, screening for certain metabolic diseases, prevention of certain respiratory illnesses, and so forth.

Unfortunately, the saving of very low birth weight infants has come with a price. A certain number grow up with developmental defects including sight, hearing, and cognitive problems requiring special education and treatment later in life.

Great advances have been made in medicine; nevertheless, as I stress throughout this book, the United States ranks way below many first world countries in neonatal mortality even though more money is spent per capita in the United States for health care than any other country. As cited earlier in this book, the World Health Organization has ranked the United States thirty-seventh in the world in regard to delivery of health care services. Nowhere is this more true than in the field of pediatrics, where our morbidity and mortality rates stand firmly at the thirty-seventh ranking. That is, we are thirty-seven behind most industrialized countries. Costs of care for pediatric patients is twice as much as in other countries, including our neighbor to the north, Canada. Causes for this rating are many, such as lack of health insurance, impoverishment, a lack of universal health care, prenatal care neglect and malnutrition, very young single mothers, drug abuse, and so forth.

One special interest to all physicians, including pediatricians, is what I like to call the fattening of America. One of every three Americans is morbidly overweight.[3] The epidemic is worsening, especially around lower economic zones where there seems to be a plethora of fast food stores. Even in affluent areas, obesity abounds. As a member of the Board of Health of Westchester County, I meet monthly with other members and one of our recurring discussions is what to do about obesity. We have health department staff going to schools, giving lectures, and handing out cartoon stories about proper eating. Some of our school districts are noteworthy for not selling soft drinks, candy, and other sugar-contaning products in their vending machines or in their lunch room cafeterias. My community of Somers leads the pack. The health department recently passed laws forbidding food cooked with transfats and laws requiring that calorie contents be posted in plain sight in fast food stores.

But this is all to no avail if the obese parents of these soon to be obese children do not change their ways. You can teach children what and what not to eat, but it is their parents who do the shopping. It is the parents who stock the house with candy, cakes, sodas, and ice cream. It is the parents who take comfort in these "comfort" foods. And it is the parents who encourage their offspring to imitate them.

One problem that confronts all physicians and perhaps pediatricians more than others is the injudicious use of antibiotics. Keep this in mind: most fevers and illnesses in kids are caused by itsy-bitsy submicroscopic germs called viruses. With few exceptions, medications have no effect on these critters. Yet, thousands of times a day, they are prescribed unnecessarily for such benign viral illnesses such as the common cold. And it is not necessarily the doctors' fault. Many parents, frightened by old-wives tales, as well as the media, have come to correlate fever with a life-threatening illness. As a consequence they expect, indeed, demand, a prescription for antibiotics.

Rather than explain that antibiotics should only be used for infections caused by bacteria, or perhaps for fear of losing the patient, an antibiotic is prescribed. Why is this bad? Well, bacteria have learned to thwart off antibiotics by changing (mutating) to other forms and have become more and more resistant to many of our most common germs. We have all heard stories about methicillin-resistant *Staphylococcus aureus* (MRSA), a form of bacteria resistant to most if not all antibiotics, and tuberculosis, strep pneumococcus, and hemophilus are further examples of these germs. By giving antibiotics needlessly, we help colonies of germs become resistant and, thus, when they are really needed, they become useless and ineffective. Experts feel that we are fast approaching a time similar to the preantibiotic era. I am sure that if you ask your pediatrician if the antibiotic he or she just prescribed was absolutely necessary, 50 percent of the time he or she would answer no.

Autism, the topic of many talk shows and recent written articles, has many parents frightened. Television loves to talk about it and Larry King has invited celebrities such as Jenny McCarthy, the ex-*Playboy* model, to vent her feelings regarding the cause. The common thought espoused by the lay press is that autism was first caused by small amounts of mercury, a preservative used in certain vaccines. When it was shown in several studies that autism actually increased or stayed the same in certain populations after the mercury was removed, the so-called experts then blamed the increased number of immunizations that children receive.[4] The cause is still unknown, although there seems to be a genetic link, perhaps acted upon by some environmental factors. There also seems to be an increase in the number of kids being labeled as autistic who previously would have been labeled as brain damaged or as having cerebral dysfunction syndrome or simply as having a speech/language delay.

What isn't in doubt is the number of children, and adults, who no longer have to worry about dying or being permanently disabled from such scourges as diphtheria, whooping cough, tetanus, polio (infantile paralysis), most meningitis types, certain pneumonias, measles, measles encephalitis, influenza, rubella (responsible for 50,000 congenital defects such as blindness, congenital heart disease and deafness in the 1960s), mumps, chickenpox, hepatitis, cervical cancer, a form of severe respiratory disease in babies born prematurely, and a form of diarrhea particularly dangerous in the first year of life. Vaccines have successfully been used to prevent such diseases. Still think shots are bad for your kids?

However, you must remember to bring your child's immunization records with you when visiting your pediatrician. Years ago, when my daughter Elyse was a toddler, the nurse showed up with syringes in each hand. "Wait a minute," my wife cried out, "Elyse is up to date with her shots." The perplexed nurse rechecked the records and, yes, there were two patients named Elyse Klein and our daughter was almost about to receive the other's shots. You should also know that all live virus vaccines have to be given subcutaneously (i.e., under the skin). These shots include measles, mumps, and rubella. Killed viruses and bacterial shots have to be given deep, into the muscle (polio, hepatitis B, diphtheria). Your pediatrician knows this, but does the nurse who is giving the shot? Lastly, regarding immunizations, your pediatrician should give you an informed consent regarding reactions one could possibly get from each vaccine. For example, pertussis vaccine can cause encephalopathy and you should know the early signs (excessive crying and fever).

Parents often question when to call the doctor. The pat answer is whenever your gut tells you that something is wrong. There is an old adage in pediatrics: "When a parent thinks the child is sick, even though the doctor doesn't, believe the mom." It is important to note that in the first three months of life, when a baby's natural ability to fight off illness is low, even minor symptoms should be taken seriously. Therefore, during this early period of time try to avoid kissing, handling by strangers, and kids with runny noses. Even a low grade fever may require hospitalizing an infant at this age.

At any age, symptoms requiring medical care include seizures, extreme lethargy, high fever, persistent diarrhea and/or vomiting, as well as difficult breathing. Possible medication overdose, poisonings, trauma, any period of unconsciousness, pallor, joint pain, and rashes complete the list. This list is certainly not inclusive, your child's physician will offer further guidance.

ADHD is another problem some parents confront. While the 2-year-old child is normally overactive and has an attention span of two seconds, how do you and the teacher handle the 8-year-old disruptive child who constantly bolts from his or her seat, is unable to follow instructions, and goes from task to task without accomplishing anything? Most experts in the field of behavioral pediatrics (yet another specialty!) rely on a multidisciplinary approach, combining pediatricians, psychologists, learning specialists, the school, and the parents. Current treatment consists of first ruling out an underlying disorder, placement in a classroom with a small number of students, less distractions, and in some cases, the use of medication.

As in all fields of medicine, you must be part of the treating team. I call this the three Q program. This requires questioning your doctor, Googling his or her response, and then questioning your doctor again. Years ago, when Lyme disease was discovered, our babysitter took our daughter to the covering doctor, as our pediatrician was off and we were away for the weekend. The babysitter rightly showed the doctor the bump on her head where she had removed an "insect." She told him that Jessica had been crying all afternoon and was covered by a rash. Well, the doctor had no clue as to the cause of the rash and fever. He did not recognize the rash and sent her home. I asked the babysitter to take Jessica to the dermatologist, who really knew his rashes. The diagnosis was promptly made and antibiotics affected the cure. A second opinion is always in order.

If it is good enough for you, it is good enough for your young loved ones. Your child's health or even life may depend upon your decisions. A patient brought her 15-year-old to me for a second opinion. The girl was a ballet student but stopped dancing because of complaints of weakness and knee pains. The pediatrician refused to do a Lyme test, despite two requests by the mother. "No, she has growing pains," said the pediatrician. It was not a big deal to do the test and it certainly was in order. The test was positive for old Lyme disease, which meant more than three months old. When we are infected, our body first produces antibodies we call immunoglobulin M (IgM). These remain in our systems for up to three months. Shortly after one month of an infection, our bodies start producing the second wave, immunoglobulin G (IgG) antibodies. Her blood had no IgM but only IgG. When I presented this to the pediatrician, he still could not be convinced, for whatever odd reason, so I treated her and she is now happily dancing. She also now has a new pediatrician.

Incidentally, it is a good policy to keep a list of your child's past immunizations with you in case another covering doctor, who might not have access to past records, has to see your child. Finally, try to stay away from emergency rooms for minor illnesses. The cost is high, the waiting periods are long, the person seeing your child is unfamiliar with him or her, and the treatment is often cursory. Besides, there may be some really sick people sitting next to you who might be contagious, drunk, or worse.

This chapter has touched only on the high spots and it is by no means comprehensive: there are many good books on child care that deserve your attention. Dr. Benjamin Spock's *Baby and Child Care* book (newly revised) is a good standard and a place to start. Avoid the junk books on medicine that are often found in pharmacies and health stories that promise you cures and state that all illness is due to a low blood sugar or a fungus that lives in your intestines. Snake oil medicine isn't dead! Step right up and buy a bottle.

PRESCRIPTION

- Bring a list of questions to each well and sick visit your child has.
- Record all of your child's immunizations for quick reference.
- Get a second opinion whenever necessary.
- Question your doctor's prescription for antibiotics regarding their necessity.

- Be sure to take your child for well visits according to the recommended schedule.
- Make sure your pediatrician washes his or her hands before your child is examined.
- Many pediatricians do office suturing as our kids are always falling and cutting themselves. Make sure a sterile technique is used (gloves and a sterile drape).
- Always be with your child, especially in a hospital setting (or have an advocate at their side). We speak about medication errors and wrong injections. Without you at your child's side, it would be easy for the child to get the wrong shot (this is covered in the section of drug errors).
- If your pediatrician is ill during a visit to the office, ask to be seen by a different doctor or reschedule.
- If your child needs surgery, try to find a pediatric surgeon, if possible.
- Seek evaluation for children who are not reaching milestones or are exhibiting symptoms of learning disorders, autism, or other psychological or mental disorders.
- Keep your children's medical records up to date.

THE PHARMACY AND PRESCRIPTION DRUGS: OR BEWARE OF THE SPOONFUL OF SUGAR THAT HELPS THE "MEDICINE" GO DOWN

It is easy to get a thousand prescriptions but hard to get one single remedy.

—Chinese Proverb[1]

I recently reviewed a malpractice claim where the charge of delay of diagnosis of a serious infection led to the patient having to undergo heart valve replacement for endocarditis. What was so striking from the beginning was the fact that the physician's assistant (PA) took a history on two separate office visits, three weeks apart. On each visit, the PA duly noted, in his own handwriting, that the patient had an allergy to ampicillin, a form of penicillin. Yet on the second visit, the PA ordered a Prev Pac (a combination of antibiotics that included ampicillin) for the eradication of unrelated intestinal bacteria. Any reviewer will know that if you start with such a blatant mistake, surely many more will follow.

According to the Institute of Medicine, at least 1.5 million patients are harmed every year from being given the wrong drugs.[2] That is an average of one person per U.S. hospital per day. And over seven thousand of those people die. Some physicians will try to undercut these numbers, saying that out of the millions of people who visit hospitals and are given drugs, this represents a small percentage. But that is simply a spin job. To use the airplane analogy again that was presented at the beginning of this book, that would be like saying that it is okay that a jumbo jet crashes every day and either seriously injures or kills many of the people on board because that represents a small percentage of all the people who fly each year. As I stated in the Introduction, if that happened, our entire airline industry would grind to a screeching halt. I am not suggesting that our medical industry stop operating until we solve these problems. But I am suggesting that we stop making excuses and rationalizations and start dealing directly with these life and death issues.

Dangerous interactions between drugs account for the majority of medical malpractice mistakes.[3] Errors and misinterpretations occur at any of the dozens of points between a drug's manufacture and a patient's receiving treatment. It is virtually impossible for a single individual to track all potential drug interactions. Therefore, there needs to be a system to do that job for us. Drug computer entry systems, which are supposed to ensure that hospital patients get the right drugs at the right dose, are used in only 6 percent of the nation's hospitals.[4] Thirty-six hospitals were studied in Colorado and Georgia, revealing that 20 percent of medicine doses were given in error, and 7 percent of these errors were harmful. To break it down further, forty potential adverse drug events occur each day in a typical 300-bed patient facility (your average hospital).[5]

Drug injuries frequently result in medical malpractice claims, which account for the highest total expenditure of any type of procedure-related injury. The 1.5 million annual drug error injuries in hospitals cost the health system $3.5 billion every year.[6] This does not include errors in doctors' offices, local pharmacies, long-term care facilities, or patients' own homes. To complicate matters, patients frequently do not inform their physicians of all the drugs that they do take. So, in terms of becoming a more proactive patient in your health care journey, it is vital that you inform your doctor of every drug, vitamin, or herbal remedy you are taking.

One significant area in the wrongful delivery of health care is the incorrect filling of prescriptions by pharmacists (wrong medicine or wrong dose) because the physician's prescription was not legible.[7] Six percent of U.S. hospital patients are hurt by medication errors that are directly linked to bad handwriting. Everyone in the health care system is to blame for this (yes, even myself).

On a recent visit to Italy one of my accompanying friends got ill, and I escorted him to the local downtown emergency room. The accommodations were stark and one could see aged pieces of hospital equipment and furniture. We braced ourselves for an unpleasant medical experience. Surprisingly, the care given was not in keeping with the surroundings. It was exemplary. Most astonishingly, the doctor typed everything on her keyboard and printed out a complete summary of her treatment (in English) as well as typewritten, computer-generated prescriptions. To our further amazement, when we asked how much we owed, we were told that the visit was free for foreigners. That is what universal health care is all about, a subject for another book.

Another important cause of medication errors is confusing information on drug labels.[8] This is especially dangerous with free drug samples that pharmaceutical detail people (drug representatives) provide physicians. Such samples are poorly controlled and do not adequately list side effects and drug interactions, which would ordinarily be explained by the pharmacist. In general, there needs to be more accountability for pharmaceutical companies. A full discourse on the pharmaceutical industry is beyond the scope of this book. Suffice it to say that the drug companies do not manage the dispensing and usage of their drugs at the highest level. Furthermore, they do not fully disclose important negative results from clinical trials.[9]

Although any one individual cannot force such changes on these big corporations, what you can do is question everything you are prescribed; make sure you understand fully what the statistics are on the use of the drug, what the clinical studies showed, and what interactions and side effects are possible. And if you do not feel as if you are getting adequate information from your doctor or pharmacist, you know what to do—Google it! Again, not everything you read on the Web will be true or accurate, but the aggregate of information will certainly give you a clearer understanding of what you are dealing with and plenty of questions to ask your doctor or pharmacist if you so desire. I have had many patients call and say that they did not take a new medicine prescribed because they looked it up on the Web and found there were just too many potential side effects. The problem is that many people stop their medications and go without anything for months before they show up at their doctor's offices and make that pronouncement. It is all right to stop medication because you either believe you are having a reaction to it or are afraid of any of the listed side effects, but you should share that with your doctor at the time you stop taking the medicine, not months later. You may have been on the medicine for a life-threatening condition and being off of it or taking some substitute may be dangerous.

More and more people are taking more and more medicines. Therefore, the incidence of medication error is soaring. Effective strategies have been known for years but ignored. Most of the chain pharmacies have centralized and computerized systems. These computers pop up adverse interactions and possible allergies, provided the patient uses the same pharmacy consistently. Often, physicians get calls from the local pharmacy informing us of possible interactions of a new prescription we had just written for a patient. Many are interactions we know about, but many are not. Recently, I gave a patient a prescription for an antibiotic to treat his pneumonia. He was on a blood thinner and the local pharmacy promptly called and informed me that this antibiotic could alter the blood-thinning drug level either up or down. I called my patient and scheduled a blood test in two days to determine the amount of drug in the blood. The morning he was due to come in for his blood level test, I received a call from his daughter that he just coughed up three or four tablespoons of blood. Sure enough, the level of the blood thinner had shot up more than triple—in just two days. That was a pretty dramatic rise in such a short period of time. But it was a quickly learned lesson for me: never give those two particular drugs together.

What is most important about this anecdote is that there are ways to prevent such incidents from occurring. I consider myself a pretty conscientious doctor but, as you can see, errors still occur because of all the constantly changing drugs and interactions. If, however, my patient had taken the proactive measure to ask his pharmacist and myself about possible drug interactions *before* taking the drug, he could have facilitated the communication sooner and prevented the experience he went through. I am not putting the blame on him at all. What I am saying is that this is a team effort. And if you, the patient, play an active part, you can avoid many of the dangerous medical mistakes this book outlines.

PRESCRIPTION

- Patients should maintain lists of all medications and dosages and bring this list each time they see their physician; include herbal remedies, vitamins, and other supplements.
- Make sure your doctor prints out the prescription legibly. In Florida it is a law.[10] Better yet, encourage your doctors to start using electronic printouts of prescriptions, like our friends in Italy.
- Become active in double checking your medication before you leave the pharmacy.

- Make sure your name, the correct medication, and the correct dosage is on the label. (Friends once visited from the Vatican and asked if I would give them their allergy shots. I looked at the vial of allergy serum and it had the name of a monsignor on the label that was entirely different from my friend's name. If even the Holy Vatican Pharmacy can make mistakes, imagine what your corner drugstore can do!)
- Have your physician explain the exact use and necessity of the medicine.
- Get in writing the name, dose, purpose, and frequency for taking the medicine.
- Discuss side effects.
- Discuss drug interactions (with other drugs, vitamins, herbs, food, and diseases).
- There is no way a doctor or nurse can get a medicine into your system without discussing it with you. (As an intern, I was asked to give a blood-thinning intravenous injection to a patient. In those days, patients were not separated as to surgical cases on one floor and medicine patients on another floor. They were all intermingled. When I entered the room and asked the first man if he was Mr. Jones, he eyed the syringe and said, "No, that's the other guy." Well the other guy got the shot and he wasn't Mr. Jones with the pulmonary embolism. He was the chief of surgery's gastrointestinal bleeder patient, Mr. Smith. I guess neither of us was too bright. Fortunately, no harm was done, but I learned how to read wrist band identifiers after that ordeal!)
- If someone comes after you with a pill or a needle, make sure they are checking your wrist band and you know exactly what that shot is for. Remember if you are in the hospital, you should have already asked your physician for a list of all medications (including injections) that you will be getting.
- Check the resources at the back of this book for reliable Web sites and agencies that can give you more information on the drugs you are taking and their possible side effects and interactions. And if all else fails, Google it!

6

VISITING THE EMERGENCY ROOM WITHOUT FEELING LIKE A BIT-PLAYER ON A TELEVISION DRAMA

"She has had no rigors or shaking chills, but her husband states she was very hot in bed last night." "The patient has no past history of suicides." "The patient refused an autopsy."

"Mrs. Jones, why didn't you call 9-11 for an ambulance?"
"My phone doesn't have an eleven."

For many, the first introduction to a hospital is through its emergency room. That is if the hospital maintains one, and if it is open twenty-four hours a day, seven days a week. So examining emergency rooms with their problems and their capabilities is crucial to good medical care. This advanced planning will show that not all emergency rooms are the same. They deal with over 100 million visits annually in the United States alone. That means that there is a lot of room for differences in procedure and, therefore, error.[1]

In recent years, there has been an overburdening of the emergency room system. This is due largely to the fact that the emergency room is the easiest place for the vast proportion of uninsured Americans to seek treatment. By varying estimates, there are well over 45 million Americans that have no health insurance. Nursing homes add to the overcrowding of emergency rooms.[2] Most of their beds are filled with chronically ill, debilitated patients who usually have no resident physician on staff. When they become ill, the head nurse calls for an ambulance to get to the nearest emergency room. Many are near death upon arrival. Further adding to the overcrowding is the ever-increasing spread of violence and the increased amount of motor vehicle accidents. The AIDS epidemic has contributed as well, as it adds millions of patients with acute, often difficult-to-treat infections. In addition to the uninsured, many welfare patients utilize the emergency room as their primary physicians, since most private practice physicians do not participate in welfare medical programs.[3]

Managed health care programs also add to the emergency room burden because most physicians, as they have seen reimbursements severely cut back, now feel forced to squeeze into their schedule as many patients as they can to make up financially for an increased portion of what they earned in years previously. Many larger group practices and multispecialty groups seem to earn 40 to 50 percent more than their smaller group counterparts and solo practitioners. This perception is a well-known source of irritation in my medical community. The larger the group, the more negotiating power they have with the HMOs, which means they have the potential to earn more money. Small groups or solo practitioners have no clout whatsoever and are forced to accept continued cutbacks by the insurance industry. In order for these doctors to make ends meet (don't forget, the cost of doing business, rent, nurse and secretary raises, and so forth continue to rise even though doctors' reimbursement rates go down), they have to see almost double the number of patients as a few years ago. Joining a large group may be more lucrative but constraining in many ways. Aside from now having an administration of a large group as your new boss, you must refer all of your patients to only those physicians in that group. Some of those specialists may be good and some may be very bad. However, because they are so busy, these doctors have no time to run to the emergency room when a patient of theirs needs them, thus placing the burden on the emergency room staff itself. Similarly, physicians make less hospital rounds to see their patients for the same reason. A new type of medical specialty, hospitalist, has aided this transformation and made a change in the doctor-patient relationship. Hospitalists are trained to treat hospitalized patients, allowing the private physicians more time at their office practices. Fashioned on the British practice system, the concept only truly works if there is daily close communication with the private physician. As specialists in the field of medicine earn more, many physicians are giving up primary care and becoming specialists. With fewer primary care physicians available, patients turn to the emergency room. Drug abusers, seasonal epidemics such as the flu, and the closing of many emergency rooms have caused overcrowding that has reached the level of a pandemic.

Budget cuts, mergers, and poor reimbursements have led to over 400 closed emergency rooms in the United States in recent years.[4] Some hospitals are under the correct belief that their emergency rooms are a gateway for the uninsured.[5] If ill enough, any patient—including illegal immigrants—is admitted, which adds a financial burden to an already financially stressed institution if they cannot pay. By a means of deterrence, many of these hospitals do not expand their staff so their facilities can keep up with the ever-increasing costs of caring for more and more indigent patients. On the converse, by keeping emergency rooms overcrowded, the quality of patient care becomes compromised. Not a good cycle to get into. Unfortunately, this is the state many of our emergency rooms find themselves in. And these are the conditions you are likely to step into when you visit the emergency room.[6]

Overcrowded emergency rooms lead to delays in service and delays in diagnosis. A thirty-minute delay in the diagnosis of an acute myocardial infarction (heart attack) will increase the chances of death by 10 percent.[7] An electrocardiogram will diagnosis a myocardial infarction only 50 percent of the time.[8] This means that patients need to be observed for longer periods of time if heart attacks are suspected. Sadly, 5 percent of patients who present to an emergency room will be sent home in error.[9] If you are sick and feel that the emergency room staff is discharging you too quickly, ask for the administrator of the hospital to intervene. They have to provide you with a patient advocate. Remember, this is your health and life we are talking about. Forget your shyness. Forget about how they might view you or what they might think about you. If you feel you are not getting your questions answered or getting the treatment you need, you must take a stand (not literally, you should stay in your bed) and speak up. Just between you and me, if you feel you need a test and they try to assure you it isn't serious, act like you are sicker than you feel. Tell them that pain in your chest *really* hurts. If you are not being taken as seriously as you should be, lean on the side of overplaying rather than downplaying your symptoms. This will usually get them to take notice and get you the tests you need.

Ray was lucky to survive a massive heart attack as he went into ventricular fibrillation in my office years ago. I do not mean that you need to be lucky to survive in my office, but that I had not had a defibrillator in my office. Fortunately, the ambulance arrived quickly as I had called for them the moment Ray walked into my office. Luckily they had been given a defibrillator just two hours previous to my call for help. On his tenth anniversary of surviving this near death experience, Ray came in the office to thank me. His wife was too sick to come out of the car. She had been in the emergency room all night long complaining of chest pain. Sure enough, after getting her out of the car, I saw that she was truly having a heart attack, similar to but not as dramatic as her husband had had ten years before. This is an example of how easy it is to miss the diagnosis of a heart attack, because of seemingly normal test results, early in the progression of such an attack. Similarly, I have testified in at least a dozen cases involving emergency room physicians and their failure to recognize the severity of patient's symptoms and the necessity of doing abdominal CT scans. The cases usually revolve around patients presenting with acute abdominal pain, even though the pain may subsequently subside during the time the patient is waiting in the emergency room. Acute pain, as will be discussed later, that subsides can be an indication of a ruptured abdominal organ (the intestines, gallbladder, etc.). CT scans can tell if an organ has ruptured or if there is an acute inflammation (appendicitis, etc.). A useful gauge would, if you rarely visit the emergency room, then you must be really sick to be there. If you feel that sick, then demand a CT scan.

Overcrowding leads to overburdening and taxes the capabilities of the treating physicians and nursing staffs.[10] That is only part of the equation. Add to this mix, potentially inept physicians and staffs (including registered nurses, licensed practical nurses, and nurse practitioners and physician's assistants). Many emergency room physicians are inexperienced, unqualified, and inadequately trained.[11] One of my friends is an obstetrics/gynecology specialist, moonlighting in the emergency room to make extra money. Another is an internist with no real training in cardiac or surgical emergencies. But these and thousands more are our frontline defense when we get ill. I know that obstetricians are great for female problems, yet they do not make good emergency room physicians, unless they get the proper training. Most of the time, these otherwise good physicians are just not prepared for the emergency room.

Furthermore, many small emergency rooms may not have specialists readily available to do the specialty work they were trained for.[12] Likewise, many may not have CT or MRI scanners or, for that matter, technicians available on a moment's notice or during the evening. Instead, they may rely on an inexperienced emergency room physician, rather than a trained radiologist, for an interpretation. Studies have shown that nearly 40 percent of CT brain scans were misread by emergency room physicians.[13] One particularly important emergency treatment, the advanced procedure of dissolving clots in acute heart attacks, requires the availability of a cardiologist within six hours of symptom onset. Dissolving clots in an acute stroke requires the availability and interpretation of a brain CT within three hours of the onset of the stroke. The unsettling fact, however, is that a large majority of our nation's emergency rooms lack these most effective treatments for strokes and heart attacks.[14]

What about disasters? How would we do in that case? An Institute of Medicine study confirmed that hospital emergency room departments are overburdened, underfunded, and ill-prepared to handle disasters.[15] This is, as already discussed, due to increasing numbers of patients who turn to emergency rooms for primary care. An ambulance is turned away from an emergency room once every minute due to overcrowding. Seventy-three percent of emergency room directors report inadequate coverage by on-call specialists in 2006 versus 67 percent in 2004.[16] This survey referred to lack of cardiology, orthopedic, and neurosurgery specialists. Reimbursement shortages in the health care industry lead to minimal staffing. Teaching hospitals now count on interns and residents to augment or replace emergency room staffs. As an intern, I am sure I contributed a few mistakes to the medical malpractice numbers, because at that point in our education we are not adequately trained or monitored.

Now take all these issues of the overburdened, understaffed emergency room and add to it the fact that the first person who greets or screens you is quite often a clerical staffer. Sometimes you are met by a rushed nurse. Certainly the clerical staffer is not trained to recognize many true emergencies. In fact, many patients are left lying on a stretcher, as their condition worsens. When you put all of this together, is it any wonder that tragedies and mistakes occur routinely in the emergency room setting? It seems as if we hear on a regular basis in news stories about patients falling over, out of their chairs (caught on security cameras), and dying because timely medical attention was not given.

So what do you do if you or a loved one has to go to the emergency room for one of these emergencies? If you have not done your homework in advance, there is not a whole lot you *can* do. And unfortunately most people are in that camp. But because you are reading this book, you are going to be prepared . . . right? So what does that look like? It looks like calling your local emergency rooms, the ones you would most likely be taken to in an emergency, and finding out *exactly* what equipment and specialists they have or have quick access to. And if you are traveling, you can find out the status of the emergency rooms in your area.

The following story strengthens my previous argument about requesting a CT scan. One case I recently testified at was about a woman who was awakened in the middle of the night by a severe pain in her abdomen. Her husband called for an ambulance and the attendant noted in his record that every time the ambulance hit a small bump in the road the patient screamed out with severe pain. By the time the emergency room physician evaluated the patient, her abdominal pain had subsided and she felt much better. The physician said it must have been an attack of gas pain, noting there were no positive findings upon his examination. Did he or the nurse speak to the ambulance technician or had they read his report, which was quite descriptive? The patient did describe the severity of the pain but the physician told her it sounded like gas and to go home and call a physician in the morning. Had he done a white blood count or what most trained physicians would do, a CT scan of the abdomen, he would have discovered that the pain was the rupturing of her intestine and the subsequent walling off by her intestinal covering (her omentum) of this impending disaster. The next day, she complained of abdominal pain to her new physician and of the severity of her symptoms the night before. A blood count was sent to a laboratory and was ready the next morning. Unfortunately for the patient, she was admitted the next morning to the same hospital with multiple abdominal abscesses and acute peritonitis. This was because of the spread of bacterially infected feces throughout her abdomen. Her white blood count from the day before was terribly elevated. No one ever took her temperature.

This next case that I testified at is illustrative of the multiple errors that usually attend a patient when the incorrect diagnosis is made and, more telling, stuck to. A middle-age woman entered the emergency room complaining of abdominal pain and diarrhea for two to three days. She was admitted with the thought that she may have had an infection of her gastrointestinal tract (gastroenteritis). No x-ray or CT scan was done on her abdomen. A white blood count was reported that evening and it was moderately elevated. The next morning, a gastroenterologist was called and noted that if the patient was not well the next morning, he would do a flexible sigmoidoscopy, looking for an infection. Cultures of her stool were ordered.

The next morning, the nurse practitioner ordered a large dose of meperidine (Demerol), an injectable narcotic, because the patient had a severe bout of abdominal pain, a nine on a ten-point scale. Two hours later, the gastroenterologist, purportedly not reading the preceding note in the chart regarding the severe pain episode, performed the procedure. His note indicated that the patient's abdomen was extremely soft before the procedure but that she had severe pain upon awakening. This is the United States of America, not a third world country! Although there may not be twenty-four-hour access to a CT scan, there is access. The poor woman had, upon admission to the hospital, a diseased intestine. The extreme pain on the second day, requiring a narcotic injection, was the rupturing of the diseased intestine. The soft abdomen followed by extreme pain of the procedure was the spreading of the infection throughout the entire abdominal cavity (some air is used in the procedure to blow the inside of the intestine away, so that the gastroenterologist can see where he is pointing the sigmoidoscope). The air just blew the covering of the intestine away, eliminating it from guarding the rupture and allowing all of that localized infection to spread.

A CT scan was ordered for the next morning. By that time, infection was everywhere and the radiologist noted the presence of gas in the patient's urinary bladder. The patient underwent emergency surgery and was placed on antibiotics and appropriate drainage of her abscesses. Unfortunately, mistakes were piled upon mistakes, otherwise she could have had a good outcome and, perhaps, never known of all the mistakes that worsened her condition, putting her face-to-face with death. No one paid attention to the gas in the bladder, even though the radiologist suspected that it could be from gas-forming bacteria. By reading all of the medical records, not one doctor involved with the case wrote that there was an abnormal finding on the CT report. No one probably read the full report or certainly did not pay any attention to the report. She was not treated for this type of bacteria nor was there any search for this type of bacteria (no culture was done). Even though she improved enough to be sent home, she still had abdominal pains and low-grade fever. Patients should not be sent home if they are still ill.

The woman died two days later with, yes, overwhelming gas-forming bacteria: *Clostridium difficile*. A week and a half prior to her emergency room visit, the patient was seen by her physician for abdominal pain (in retrospect, acute diverticulitis) and was given antibiotics, which did not adequately treat her diseased intestine but did cause the diarrhea. *Clostridium difficile* is a bacterium that lives in the intestine (their numbers are small because their growth is limited by the millions of colonies of other hardier bacteria). When taking an antibiotic, many of the hardier bacteria will become susceptible and die, leaving the clostridia to grow to its heart's content, thus causing diarrhea! If you develop diarrhea while taking or after just finishing antibiotics, the first thing to be concerned with should be . . .? Yes, you are getting it, clostridial infection of the intestines. Why this information was not culled out by the emergency room physician, I do not know. There is a cure for *C. difficile*, but the patient's physicians did not suspect it and were not thinking of it, even though they were prewarned by the radiologist. These are true cases of ordinary people dying, just trying to get well.

It is important to remember that the first person to greet you in the emergency room will usually be an admitting clerk. You are responsible for drawing an accurate picture for the emergency staff. Do not make the mistake of downplaying your symptoms for fear of having something really wrong with you or for fear of looking bad. If you do, you will more than likely be put on a long waiting list, only to be seen after all the others. If you really are having an acute episode, time is very critical for stopping the event from causing further damage. After signifying that you are acutely ill, make sure you let them know everything that is pertinent. If you are having chest pain, it is important for them to know that your father died of a heart attack. Is there diabetes or cancer in your family? It is a good idea to carry a little medical history with your family history as well. At a time of emergency, many of us are not really thinking clearly and find it difficult to give an accurate history. If a patient comes in my office for a visit and is accompanied by a spouse, I encourage that mate to stay during the interview phase, especially if the patient is a male (they tend to forget or belittle everything). How often, even in my office (where there isn't an emergency) will the patient answer no to a question and the spouse interject with just the opposite answer? That white coat syndrome and anxiety due to illness can sure fog one's thinking process. It is similar to a study of a class of, get this, criminologists. During the class, there was some screaming and yelling as a "perpetrator" ran toward the teacher's desk and ran out again. When asked to identify what the intruder looked like, almost no one got it correct. The trauma of the intrusion tainted everyone's memory temporarily.

Your social history is also important. Do you smoke? Drink or do drugs? Now is not the time to be discreet. Let it all out. There is an increased incidence of heart disease in drug abusers. When does the pain occur? All the time? Only with twisting motions, deep breathing? Is it increased with exertion? Does it occur after you eat or have eaten something specific? Are there associated symptoms; backache, abdominal pain, shortness of breath? Is there tenderness to the touch, fever, cough, sweating? Did the pain occur suddenly and acutely or did it come about gradually? Was there trauma? (I remember seeing a patient in the emergency room who had chest pain and thought that she was having a heart attack. The pain however, was similar to a pulled muscle or strain. I asked if she had hurt herself in an accident or fall. Then she remembered that awfully tight bear hug her husband had given her the night before.)

Relate your symptoms as clearly and concisely as you can. Do not try to do a marathon of explanations, as that will lull the most conscientious physician to sleep. Physicians are like scientists, and scientific minds like their histories to be short and concise and most of all devoid of rambling. But we need all the information possible. A busy and tired physician may forget to ask all the right questions. He or she may be too tired to direct the questioning and fall prisoner to rambling. Obviously, missing the opportunity to get the information needed will keep him or her from thinking of the proper diagnosis. Without thinking of the diagnosis, it will never be made. And if it is never made, or made incorrectly, well . . . you know what happens then.

To further prepare you for dealing with specific ailments when going to the emergency room, the following sections present some of the most common concerns and possible underlying causes.

CHEST PAINS

Chest pain can obviously be caused by anything in the chest. Starting from the outside and working our way inward, one encounters the skin. Herpes zoster (shingles) starts out as a burning, tingling sensation with the skin becoming sensitive. This occurs on only one side of the body and will follow one nerve root on that part of the body. After two days, pain will start, and is followed in three to four days with a blisterlike rash. It is the same type of feeling of a fever or sun sore on the lips. The appearance of the rash and pain syndrome can be aborted by promptly taking the appropriate antiviral medication.

Deeper in the tissue layer, pain can be caused by a virus, coxsackie B or Bornholm disease. Sometimes the pain will be accompanied by a severe tightness around the chest (devil's grip) and can mimic an acute heart attack. Viral blood antibody studies, although timely, will prove the presence of acute herpes zoster and coxsackie B infection. Breast infection and some unusual virulent breast cancer will cause localized chest pain, but these are obvious. Lyme disease can cause chest pain and is usually associated with a characteristic rash.

Costochondritis is a localized pain at the area where one's ribs are attached to the sternum cartilage. It can be quite tender and hurts when touched. There are muscles between each rib that allow our chest to expand and deflate. These muscles can get stretched when wrenched or from deep coughing. There is usually localized tenderness.

Pinched nerves from the spinal column (from arthritis or disc disease) will cause pain, but the pain will usually follow along one rib (which could be on both sides of the chest, i.e., the seventh rib on the right and left). These nerves leave the spinal cord and traverses through the chest, running underneath the rib. There is a special groove under the rib, allowing room for the nerve.

The gallbladder as well as all the other organs under the diaphragm (liver, spleen, and intestine) can cause chest pain. Gastritis, ulcer disease, esophageal ailments, and gastroesophageal reflux disease (GERD) are all frequent causes of chest pain that can worry someone enough to seek medical evaluation. My patient and dear friend was taken to the emergency room by ambulance because of acute pain in his upper midchest. The pain was cardiac sounding, but all of his tests were normal. When he told me that he had eaten at another friend's home, I immediately knew the diagnosis. The other friend loves ice cream and whipped cream and, sure enough, that is what was served for dessert. These are some of the types of food that can trigger a gallbladder attack. As suspected, an immediate ultrasound (not a CT scan) confirmed an inflamed gallbladder. (This is one reason why it is good to be friendly with your doctor. This gives insight into your likes and dislikes and, aside from knowing what you eat, can be suggestive of what ails you.)

Diseases of the lungs are next in line. The lungs are organs that are covered with a plastic wrap–like membrane called the pleura. The pleura can become inflamed by infection, embolism, rarely malignancy, and from trauma. The symptom of pleurisy is chest pain, worsened by taking a deep breath. Be careful not to jump to the conclusion that you have pleurisy because of pleuritic pain (pain upon deep breathing), as musculoskeletal pain can also worsen with deep breathing.

Pulmonary embolism is often associated with pleuritic pain and is some-times accompanied by a tender breast or chest wall. The embolism has to come from an inflamed vein (usually from the calf), and that is why your calves have to be checked when trying to diagnose the cause of chest pain. Calves become thrombosed (clotted) when the legs have not moved for a prolonged period (being in a hospital bed, long car, train, or airplane trip).

Infection of the lung or bronchial tree is one of the most frequent causes of chest pain. These upper respiratory infections are probably the most common cause of emergency room visits for chest discomfort. Malignancy of the lung similarly can be a cause of chest pain. Rupture of small por-tions or blebs of the lung tissue can occur. These are due to weakening of that portion of the lung by prior infection or by congenital defects. This is a not uncommon cause of chest pain, feeling like pleuritic pain and ac-companied by shortness of breath.

The heart is covered, similar to the lungs, with a plastic wrap–like mem-brane, the pericardium. Pericarditis (inflammation of the covering of the heart) is caused by infection, embolization, coronary artery disease, and, rarely, malignancies.

When people have chest pain, they immediately concern their thoughts with coronary artery disease. And well they should. Coronary artery disease is one of the leading causes of hospitalization for adults. It is the clogging of the blood vessels that feed the heart. But prompt diagnosis of an acute or underlying coronary problem can often forestall or reverse a major event. There are some patients who are so fearful of having coronary artery dis-ease that they deny its existence. I once interviewed a patient and asked him why he was there that day. He answered, "My wife wants to know why I am having chest pain." Another patient, B. J., came in complaining of having a sore throat. After examining him and telling him that his throat looked fine, I started to leave the room. B. J. suddenly spoke up, "Excuse me, but why did I get chest pain while I was lifting up the garbage cans this morning?" Sure enough, B. J. was having a heart attack, but was so fearful of the possibility that he almost did not mention it.

Murmurs are signs of leakage through a heart valve. Physicians listen to these to see if there are changes on existing murmurs or if there is a new murmur developing. This occurs in heart valve infections, heart failure, hypertension, or pulmonary disease. Once the emergency room physician called me regarding a patient who happened to be a local dentist. John was having acute front and back chest pain. The patient was found to have a murmur by the emergency room doctor and the doctor wanted to know whether it was preexisting. I had never found a murmur previously and this was a tip-off that the patient was undergoing a dissection of his aortic artery. Certain murmurs (i.e., mitral valve prolapse) can be associated with chest pain.

After listening to the history, most diagnoses (90 percent) can be made. Then there is the examination and the laboratory for backup confirmation and enlightenment for the other 10 percent. Vital signs must always be taken as well as a good physical examination. Chest pain always warrants basic blood work (complete blood cell count [CBC] to see if there is an infection). The heart has enzymes that are released into the bloodstream upon damage to the individual heart cell. Measurement of these enzymes by blood testing is also essential. CT scan imaging will determine if there is trauma to the rib cage, pulmonary embolism, pleuritic fluid, cardiac fluid, pneumonia, ruptured lung, malignancy, and dissection of the aorta. Serial cardiograms will help detect active heart disease (something occurring at that specific moment in time) but will not tell whether there is underlying clogging of the arteries. If there is suspicion that you have coronary disease that is not being revealed by enzymes in the blood or changes in serial cardiograms, then a nuclear or echo stress test should be performed. But do not let them schedule one weeks down the road, insist on one immediately.

Sometimes stress tests are falsely negative (as well as falsely positive). Stress tests will only be positive if 70 percent of a coronary blood vessel is clogged. One could potentially have serious underlying coronary vascular disease and have a normal stress test. If the story sounds strong enough for coronary artery disease, then the thought of a cardiac angiogram should be discussed. A recent patient had chest pain while walking around the track for her daily exercise. I thought for sure that she had coronary artery disease. Her nuclear stress test turned out normal, and it took an hour for me to convince her to go the extra step and get an angiogram. The angiogram revealed that Rose had triple vessel disease (major clogging of three coronary arteries) and stenting was performed on the spot.

Should everyone entering the emergency room with chest pain wind up with a chest x-ray, CT scan, serial electrocardiogram, and stress testing? If the symptoms sound right, if you have a significant family history, if you smoke, have underlying diseases, or are really sick, you had better be ready to defend yourself. Again, we are not living in a third world country. The modern testing methods of CTs, electrocardiograms, and stress testing are available in most communities. Although I discuss the misreading and misinterpretation of these tests as major causes of maiming and death in our country, not doing the appropriate testing is a common cause of medical malpractice death.[17] That is death by not making the correct diagnosis, because of not having all the facts to do so. Before you have the facts, you have to think about what the alternatives are. Then you will know which tests have to be done. You must demand a differential list of diagnoses that could cause your problem, then have the physician tell you why you don't have this or that diagnosis.

One of my patients was admitted to the local hospital, while I was on vacation, for significant chest pain. He was observed for two days and all of his tests were normal. His stress test was also normal and he was sent home. His insurance company was refusing to pay for his two-day hospitalization, stating that one day would have been sufficient, especially since his stress test was normal. Upon return from vacation, I interviewed James and realized that he rarely came in for illnesses. I commented that he must have been in real severe pain to go to the emergency room. He said, "Doc, that was the worst chest pain that I ever had, it really took my breath away." That classic line made me send him off for an immediate angiogram. He had one main coronary vessel that was nearly closed, which failed to show up with serial enzymes and cardiograms, as well as a nuclear stress test. Knowing a patient and listening carefully to the severity of his symptoms is what saved James's life. Aside from Rose and James, there have been at least twenty patients over the past three or four years who had "the story." They passed stress testing with flying colors but had a story for strong or unusual pain that contradicted the normal stress test. It is unfortunate, but it happens all too often. The doctor must know his or her patient and be able to tell the measure of discomfort. If the story fits, the "jury" has to order a catheterization. Catheterization has developed into a safe and acceptable modality for diagnosing the existence of coronary disease. Years ago, I sent a patient, Anthony, for a stress test. He was 38 and had had chest pain. Unfortunately, his stress test was normal. It was during that period of time that cardiac catheterization was in its infancy. It was unheard of in those days to really question a negative stress test and go on to doing a catheterization. Anthony died two days later of a massive heart attack, sadly, for him and his family, and sadly for me, as even we physicians are truly saddened when someone needlessly dies. That is one of the reasons for this book. With learning from experience as a guide, I am now very aggressive with patients with chest pain in today's environment.

There is an obvious importance in promptly diagnosing coronary artery disease. Acute heart attacks are life-threatening and can often be reversed by a procedure called thrombolysis. This is the introduction of a clot-dissolving chemical into the circulatory system. The clot, which is blocking the coronary artery and causing the heart attack, is thusly dissolved. Not every emergency room is equipped with this medicine (or many not have an available cardiologist to administer it). That is where pre-illness due diligence pays off. Furthermore, there is only a small window of time between the onset of symptoms and effective medication administration. The medication has to be administered one hour after symptoms of a stroke occur to reverse the stroke (one must first prove that the stroke is caused by a clot and not a bleeding or ruptured blood vessel by doing a CT scan). To reverse a heart attack, the medicine has to be administered within six hours of the onset of symptoms. So the quicker the diagnosis is made, the better the outcome. The latest controversy regarding treatment of an ongoing heart attack involves the recent evidence that angiography and stenting of the affected coronary artery may be more beneficial than thrombolysis therapy. This would require that the patient be transferred and get an angiogram within that same six-hour time frame.

DIZZINESS

Dizziness is often a common reason for adults to visit an emergency room. Although it may become incapacitating and disabling, dizziness does not usually signal a serious or life-threatening illness. By definition dizziness describes a number of subjective symptoms, which the patient may describe as feelings of lightheadedness, floating, wooziness, giddiness, confusion, disorientation, or loss of balance. Causes may stem from a variety of failures of equilibrioception, hypotension, cerebral hypoxia, or a reaction to environmental chemicals or drugs. My 3-year-old son Matthew loves to spin around the room until he feels dizzy and falls to the ground. He obviously thinks that is a great way to entertain himself; however, if it happened to adults, it would not be fun at all. There is a distinct difference to physicians in the various descriptions of dizziness.

Vertigo

Vertigo is a specific term physicians use to describe the sensation of having the room spin about you (the sensation of spinning) and is often accompanied by nausea and vomiting (the body's reaction to spinning). Vertigo usually derives from two separate sources: the inner ear and the central nervous system.

Commonly known inner-ear maladies are Menière's disease, labyrinthitis, and benign positional vertigo (BPV). The latter occurs usually in later life and can sometimes mimic a tiny stroke (or transient ischemic attack [TIA]).

Menière's disease is caused by the excessive buildup of fluid in one's inner ear. It usually affects adults. The symptoms show themselves with sudden episodes of spinning, which lasts for thirty to sixty minutes. Patients usually complain of buzzing or ringing in the ear and a feeling of fullness in the head, with some mild hearing loss.

Inflammation of the inner ear such as labyrinthitis, or acute vestibular neuronitis, is characterized by a sudden, intense spinning sensation, which may persist for several days. Patients are usually nauseous or vomiting and may have a feeling of being off-balance, requiring bed rest.

BPV is a disease with intense, short episodes of a spinning sensation associated with the changing of one's head position. It can occur in drivers, as they turn behind them to see traffic, or when we turn over in bed. The turning of the head initiates the syndrome.

Vertigo from migraine headaches can be accompanied by a visual "aura" or what many patients describe as dizziness or severe vertigo.

Acoustic neuromas are benign growths in the inner ear. They are attached to the vestibular nerve and can be accompanied by loss of balance, hearing loss, ringing in the ear, and of course, vertigo.

Rarely, serious underlying illnesses can be accompanied by vertigo (brain hemorrhage, stroke, multiple sclerosis), but these account for a minority of emergency room dizziness visits.

Disequilibrium

The term disequilibrium applies to a sensation of being off balance or unsteadiness and is usually not associated with nausea or vomiting. Patients usually have frequent falls. Inner ear (vestibular) abnormalities can cause a feeling of "floating" or unsteadiness, especially in the dark. Failing vision or peripheral nerve damage (due to aging or diseases such as diabetes) of the lower extremities can cause difficulties in maintaining one's balance, especially in the elderly. Various medications can cause a loss of balance. One immediately thinks of narcotics, but a common side effect for the antibiotic doxycycline, used for the treatment of Lyme disease, is loss of balance.

PRESYNCOPE

Syncope is the term we use for fainting or passing out. Presyncope, or lightheadedness, is accompanied by the feeling of faint and muscular weakness, but not actually passing out. This last group of illnesses, which comprise presyncope, does not originate from the inner ear or from central nervous system diseases. It is usually caused by cardiovascular diseases or orthostatic hypotension (lightheadedness due to a significant drop of one's blood pressure).

In order to lead our examiner in the right direction, we (and hopefully the doctor) should know these differences. Are you lightheaded, off balance, is the room spinning? Are you nauseous or vomiting? There is a subtle difference between having the sensation of one's head floating and holding on for dear life as the room spins around you. Many patients will have some of the causes mentioned above, however, there are many patients who show up at the emergency room with panic attacks, which can be associated with lightheadedness or dizziness. Many of these patients continue further into hyperventilation (abnormal rapid breathing usually associated with anxiety attacks).

HEADACHES

There are two types of head pain: primary and secondary. Secondary headaches are caused by some associated illness, which may be quite serious. Primary headaches are limited to tension headaches, migraines, and cluster headaches.

Primary Headaches

The most common forms of headaches are due to tension and are called tension headaches. They are often described as a band of pressure encircling the head with the most intense part of pain over the eyebrows. They are usually mild and affect both sides of the head. Migraines, the second most common form of primary headaches, are always recurrent. They are intense, throbbing (pounding), and affect just one side of the head. Cluster headaches come in groups (or clusters), which last for weeks or months, then go away for prolonged periods of time. This pain also occurs on one side of the head and recurs a few times during the day.

Secondary Headaches

Secondary headaches can have numerous causes, although you may not know immediately that the headache you are feeling is being caused by something other than a primary reason. Typically, however, headaches that are caused by secondary reasons tend to be much more extreme, much more frequent, or produce other neurological symptoms (speech problems, partial paralysis, etc.). Migraines can also cause associated symptoms, such as light sensitivity and eyesight problems. Here is a list of some of the causes of secondary headaches:

- Brain tumor
- Epidural hematoma (due to rapid collection of arterial blood secondary to head trauma and usually is associated with loss of consciousness)
- Subdural hematomas (blood under the covering of the brain, secondary to a ruptured blood vessel). This usually occurs in elderly people who have fallen and then develop changes in personality and weakness. Since they can occur gradually, many elderly may not recollect falling.
- Stroke (characterized as severe headaches associated with seizure or coma). This is also associated with paralysis (or weakness) of one side of the body. There may or may not be speech defects, drooping of the mouth, or unexplained falling. We now call strokes brain attacks, to highlight the severity and similarity to heart attacks.

The importance of identifying a stroke in progress cannot be overstated. Eighty percent of strokes are caused by a clot in a cerebral artery. These clots can be dissolved if diagnosed within a three-hour timeframe. The use of MRIs enables a doctor to distinguish between the 80 percent caused by clots (which are treatable) and the 20 percent caused by bleeding. When researching emergency rooms in your area, you must find out if there is 24/7 coverage for MRIs and their reading, but also if there is clot-dissolving therapy available. This is important for strokes as well as heart attacks.[18]

Headaches from infections are a common cause of emergency room visits. Lyme disease and ehrlichiosis are quite common causes of severe headaches (and hence emergency room visits) in my area. These headaches can be so severe that I have often heard my patients state "If I had a gun, I would shoot myself!" Infections such as meningitis and sinusitis are also causes of visits.

Uncommon causes of headache such as subarachnoid bleeding (ruptured aneurysms), temporal arteritis, and sudden onset of severely elevated blood pressure must be kept in mind to prevent blindness or death.

Making sure the doctor gets a full history is very important in evaluating headaches. But many patients may have to undergo CT scans, MRIs, or even lumbar puncture to rule out life-threatening diseases. Blood testing can help distinguish infection (Lyme titers, CBC) and vasculitis (sedimentation rates for temporal arteritis). Meningitis usually is associated with fever and neck stiffness as well as rapid mental deterioration. CT scans and MRIs will detect tumors and the various types of cranial bleeding and strokes.

When reporting to the emergency room with head pain, do not understate your pain or symptoms. In fact, I suggest you lean on the side of overstating them, of being a little dramatic. In the potential chaos of the emergency room environment, it might be the thing that gets you the proper attention—and the necessary and timely tests.

ABDOMINAL PAIN

When evaluating abdominal pain, one should take the same approach as that of chest pain. Pain can emanate from the skin. Rashes, herpes zoster, and pinched nerves can cause pain, tingling, hypothesia (loss of sensation), or burning. Again, pinched nerves and herpes zoster are usually found on one side of the body and follow the nerve root under the ribs. As an example, a pinched nerve in the upper back or the chest will radiate around to the sides of the chest, following the rib and cause a radicular route, to the front of the abdomen, far down, below the belly button.

Diseased upper abdominal structures can cause chest pains. Similarly, diseased lower abdominal and pelvic structures can cause pain in the upper abdomen. In fact, the usual first sign of appendicitis is that of upper abdominal pain, before it ultimately settles in the right lower abdomen. Pain under the lower ribs can be caused by breaking or fracture of the cartilage that connects the floating ribs to the chest bone.

Muscle layers crisscross our abdomens. These layers can have weak points between them, which can separate. This is caused either by heredity or from continued intraabdominal pressure. A hernia is the protrusion through a portion of the peritoneum by an intraabdominal organ (piece of intestine). This intestine pushes through this weakened wall or muscle separation. It can occur on any part of the abdomen and range in size from tiny to very large. Localized pain on any part of the abdomen may be from a hernia, which may be too small to be seen.

A plastic wrap–like substance, the peritoneum, encases the intestine, abdominal, and pelvic organs. Inflammation of the peritoneum (peritonitis) usually comes from some catastrophe inside this covering. This condition requires prompt and immediate attention, as acute peritonitis is a true medical emergency. This is called an acute abdomen. The condition connotes an inflamed or infected intestine, or an abdominal or pelvic organ, such as an appendix. Or it can signify something more ominous such as a ruptured organ or intestine or an embolization (clot) to any of those structures.

The gallbladder and kidneys can become blocked by a stone, which usually causes severe pain. Gallbladder pain usually occurs in the right upper abdomen, but as my friend Joey can attest, it can shoot pain up to the mid- and, rarely, the left chest. Kidney pain is usually on one side (the flank) and kidney stones cause severe intermittent pain. Pain of a kidney stone only occurs when the stone starts moving, trying to pass itself down the urinary tract.

The intestines twist and turn during normal digestion. These twists and turns can sometimes cause the intestine to get caught in a certain position, especially if there is scar tissue from a previous surgery. The elder intestine can also suffer from a lack of blood supply (ischemia, similar to coronary artery insufficiency). This can cause heart attack–like pain in the abdomen, which is often associated with rectal bleeding. As the intestine ages, small out-pouches (diverticula) appear. They have been compared to the bulge on a spare tire. These bulges can become inflamed (diverticulitis) and can even rupture. Although not proven scientifically, in my experience attacks can often be initiated by eating nuts or corn. The pain often occurs in the left lower abdomen but can also occur on the right side. Infections or inflammations inside the colon (enteritis, food poisoning, ulcerative colitis, Crohn's disease) are frequent causes of abdominal pain. Pelvic organs also cause acute and chronic pain syndromes.

As one can see, the proper diagnosis of the cause of abdominal pain can be quite complex. The old adage of "to cut is to cure" no longer holds. Unless one is bleeding to death, surgery usually has to await the confirmation of the right, but prompt, diagnosis.

The progression of symptoms is important. Did they start gradually or acutely? Where did the pain start? Was it accompanied with sweats, chills, or fever? Were they shaking chills? Acute infections usually are accompanied by severe shaking chills (indicating bacteria entering the bloodstream). The chills notify us that a fever is soon to follow, which is one of the body's defense mechanisms to fight off the bacteria. This is common in urinary tract or gallbladder infections, which spill from those systems into the bloodstream (sepsis).

What medicines, tonics, or herbal remedies were consumed? Had you had them before? Nonsteroidal anti-inflammatories, aspirin, ibuprofen (Advil), and other such drugs can cause erosion of the gastric mucosa. Medicines for osteoporosis can cause severe abdominal complaints. Doxycycline (a form of tetracycline used for acne and Lyme disease) can cause severe burning of the esophagus. Does the pain go away with antacids? In the old days, a patient with midchest or abdominal pain would be given an immediate dose of four ounces of an antacid to see if the pain was gastrointestinal in origin. Was the pain acutely severe, then went away (remember the lady with the ruptured intestine)? Is the pain continuous or only when you move? Kidney stones cause continuous pain while they are trying to travel through the ureter (renal passage). Back pain from a herniated disc, on the other hand, usually hurts only when one moves. What was the time relationship between the onset of symptoms and when you ate a suspected meal? Where were you traveling? It is obvious if you were in a third world country and developed abdominal pain and diarrhea. However, many resort areas, including ski resorts in our own country, have faulty water systems. Many a domestic vacationer has come down with *Escherichia coli* (*E. coli*) or intestinal parasites.

My wife and I were vacationing in Maui. While she was just finishing her lunch, which was the hotel restaurant's special of the day, grilled mahi mahi, she started developing cramps in her abdomen. About ten minutes later, she became nauseous and vomited. This was followed by numbness, then by copious diarrhea. Not a pleasant sight and, for her, a horribly frightening ordeal. She then broke out with a bright red rash over her entire body and her pulse shot up to 150 beats per minute. Food poisoning is never that rapid, but the locals refer to this episode as the mahi mahi flush. Improperly refrigerated mahi mahi causes the release of histamine from the muscles of the fish. This abnormality is not recognizable by inspection or smell. The fish looks and tastes normal, but a mouthful of this histamine concoction will cause a severe allergic reaction, as occurred in my wife. Fortunately, we travel with cortisone and diphenhydramine (Benadryl), and her "near death experience" lasted only two hours.

POSSIBLE EXAMINATION PROCEDURES AND TESTS

After your vital signs, your physician should be listening to your bowel sounds (the intensity of the gurgling). Increased bowel sounds occur in food poisoning, infections, or inflammations within the bowel walls. Early in an intestinal obstruction, they will be hyperactive (increased), trying to unblock stool passage. Hypoactive (decreased) or absent bowel sounds can connote a ruptured organ, peritonitis, or a complete blockage. After abdominal or pelvic surgery, our intestines go to sleep (ileus) and stop their peristaltic (churning) motion. It is nature's way of allowing them to heal. That is one reason why patients cannot eat or drink after such surgeries. Otherwise the food or liquid will just lie there. And that is why the nurse or physician will keep listening to our bowel sounds for a sign of gas. I always thought it humorous that after surgery is the only time when it is socially acceptable for a person to pass gas. That is why patients are always asked "Did you pass gas yet?"

The physical examination will include looking at the skin for rashes. The other day, a 21-year-old man came in with scratch marks over one side of his abdomen. "You know those fatty small tumors you told me I had? Well, they just became extremely itchy!" His scratch marks were deep but were nowhere near his fatty lumps. They followed his nerve roots on that one side. His diagnosis was a prelude to an attack of shingles. A woman came in with abdominal pain and weight loss. When she showed me her abdomen, there was a protuberance of her lower abdomen, despite the weight loss. Her diagnosis was a tumor. The trained eye and hand can see and feel lumps and bumps as well as the tautness of the abdominal muscles. If the abdominal muscles are hard and painful to the touch, it is peritonitis until proven otherwise. Not only will there be tenderness, but if the physician presses on the other side of the abdomen and then quickly releases the pressure, the patient will feel extreme pain where the disease is. By the way, if you are ticklish during the abdominal examination, place your hand on top of the examining physician's hand. He may think you are weird but you won't laugh, as it is hard to tickle yourself.

Rectal and pelvic examinations are to some degrading. But every piece of information aids in the proper diagnosis. Is there stool in the rectum? If none, there could be an obstruction. Is there microscopic (occult) blood present? How high up is the blood? What color is the stool? Black stool can come from upper gastrointestinal bleeding, but it can also come from eating spinach or drinking bismuth (Pepto-Bismol). Is the stool very light? This suggests liver disease. If there is diarrhea, are there white blood cells present? This is a sign of infection or colitis. Is the stool sent for laboratory studies? The rectal examination can frequently tell if there is cancer present. Many colon cancers occur within finger reach of the anus. The rectal examination will also access the prostate. Vaginal examinations are so important in the evaluation of abdominal pain. If they are not done, then there is something wrong with the methodology of the examining physician.

Laboratory testing for white blood cells in the serum (infection) and for red blood counts will indicate bleeding. If the patient is Hispanic or African American, a hemoglobin electrophoresis should be done for undiagnosed abdominal pain. Patients with sickle cell disease can have acute abdominal crisis. Urine analysis should be done for abdominal pain. Many times urinary tract infection or kidney stones can cause unusual abdominal pain. Sugar in the urine can suggest diabetes, which is a cause of diarrhea and abdominal pain. CT scanning of the abdomen and pelvis with and without contrast material is one of the most helpful tools at our disposal. If diverticulitis or appendicitis is suspected, a CT scan will usually confirm its presence or absence. Years ago, surgeons just jumped in if appendicitis was suspected because one did not want to miss a hot appendix. Today, we can confirm the diagnosis and thereby avoid unnecessary surgery. Laboratory testing is very helpful. Certain enzymes are released into the bloodstream when certain abdominal organs are inflamed. We measure levels of amylase, lipase, and liver function enzymes (bilirubin, gamma glutamyl transferase [GGT], aspartate aminotransferase [AST], alanine aminotransferase [ALT], alkaline phosphatase, etc.), which points our attention to the pancreas, liver, and gallbladder. Seventy percent of duodenal ulcers are now found to be associated with the presence of the bacteria *Helicobacter pylori*. Antibodies to this bacterium are found in the blood and this has now become a common diagnostic tool. The fact is, there are many diagnostic tools immediately at our disposal. Every major center has not only CT and MRI scanning, but abdominal angiograms, hepatobiliary iminodiacetic acid (HIDA) scanning (for gallbladder activity), and endoscopic retrograde cholangiopancreatography (ERCP) for pancreatic diseases. Endoscopy and sigmoid/colonoscopy are also part of our diagnostic armamentarium. (Colonoscopies are not indicated in suspected acute diverticulitis or perforated bowels, but need to be done months later.)

A friend of mine once commented that the police are like a double-edged sword. One needs protection, but at times one needs protection from the protection. Medicine, similarly, presents the same irony. Mistakes happen during the normal course of our encounters with patients and have to be recognized immediately before they spin out of control and someone is harmed. Although we have no control of when illness strikes, it is better to avoid emergency rooms in the busy winter months. Generally, emergency rooms are busy all day on Mondays and during the evenings of Fridays and Saturdays. Especially avoid teaching hospitals during the month of July, when training staffs rotate or just start. Summer horror stories aren't just fiction. The adjusted mortality rate rises 4 percent in July and August for the average teaching hospital. That is, eight to fourteen more deaths occur at major teaching hospitals than would normally without the staff turnover.[19] If I were a patient in the emergency room, I would have no problem saying to the examining physician, "With all the horror stories one hears about medical mistakes in emergency rooms and hospitals in general, I'm quite frightened to be here." I would suggest you consider saying something similar. That would serve notice and put the physician on heightened alertness, perhaps an "orange alert." At the very least, it could snap the doctor out of the automatic routine and increase the chances of him or her actually thinking through your case thoroughly. You could probably get the same effect if you drop in the line, "By the way, my brother is a very famous malpractice attorney!"

So what does all this mean for you, the proactive patient? The most important thing to get out of this section is not necessarily a diagnosis of your particular ailment (if you have one now)—and certainly not a *fear* of emergency rooms—but rather a sense of the many possibilities that your symptoms can represent and the many options for diagnosis of them. Understanding these issues, knowing the emergency room conditions, and having a basic working knowledge of your body will allow you to ask more informed questions, give more descriptive details about symptoms, and, yes, even suggest possible diagnoses to your doctor.

It is your body, after all. Why shouldn't you know it better than anyone else? Why shouldn't you have a working knowledge of how this most precious part of your life operates? For too long the medical establishment has made patients feel as if they were dependent on doctors and experts to understand their bodies, their health, and how to get and stay well. It has sown a myth that doctors are godlike or superior and hold the answers to your well-being. And it has created an epidemic of uninformed, intimidated patients who are either too afraid or, to be blunt, too ignorant about their symptoms, causes, and conditions to take an active role in their healing. Fortunately, that won't be you anymore.

PRESCRIPTION

- Find out what equipment is available in your local emergency room. If you are traveling, locate the closest emergency room and find out what is available there.
- Find out how many physicians and nurses work each shift per patient volume.
- Find out if there is a reliance on physician's assistants and nurse practitioners. (They are knowledgeable but not as much as physicians, otherwise they would be called physicians.)
- Inquire whether the physicians in the emergency room are board certified in emergency medicine.
- Ask if there is twenty-four-hour access to CT, MRI, and attending radiologists to read them.
- If you present with abdominal pain, demand a CT scan if it is not ordered.
- Acute chest pain may be due to heart problems, lung infections, and, not as uncommonly as one would think, pulmonary embolisms, espe-

cially if the pain is increased with a deep breath. This condition can be diagnosed with a CT scan of the lungs.

- You know when treatments are rushed or inattentive or haphazard. If you are sick, ask for a second opinion or ask for the hospital administrator to intervene. (Don't take your treatment lying down! I mean, you may actually have to lie down for treatment, but don't stand for just any treatment!)

- Find out what subspecialists are available on a moment's call (cardiologists, neurosurgeons, chest surgeons, etc.).

- Don't hesitate to remind the on-call emergency room doctor of your concerns, considering all the errors made in emergency rooms and hospitals. It can quickly wake them up!

- Avoid using the emergency room for regular office visits; you will wait forever, get substandard care in many cases, and clog their system with unnecessary visits.

- If possible, avoid emergency rooms in July (that is when the new physicians arrive in training hospitals).

- If possible, avoid emergency rooms on Mondays, as well as Friday and Saturday evenings. That is when they are the busiest.

II

MAJOR DISEASES AND
LONG-TERM ISSUES

7

A REAL HEART-TO-HEART ABOUT CARDIAC CARE

By the time he was admitted, his rapid heart had stopped and he was feeling better.

Patient has chest pain if she lies on her left side for over a year.

—Diagnoses as written up on charts

Coronary artery disease is the leading cause of death and morbidity in the United States. It claims the lives of over one-half million Americans annually.[1] The diagnosis can be difficult, given the inaccuracies of stress testing (both false-positive and false-negative results occur commonly). Furthermore, many stress tests are interpreted as normal by cardiologists when abnormal findings are present. Nuclear scans obtained while stress testing can appear normal, but when accompanied by electrocardiogram changes that are abnormal, the cardiologist should be wary. According to prior teaching, if the nuclear scan was normal and the electrocardiogram was abnormal, the test was deemed normal. I have questioned many of these "normal" reports with the cardiologists and have often sent the patient for a different type of test to make sure there wasn't any underlying disease. In fact, we now know that 10 to 30 percent of these negative/positive (scan negative/electrocardiogram positive) are shown to really be positive.[2] To avoid these pitfalls, more reliance should be placed on stress echocardiograms, which rely on abnormal wall motion as an indicator of disease, regardless of whether the electrocardiogram is positive or negative.[3] As you will see in this chapter, it sure has paid off for me. This negative report by the cardiologist leads patients to believe that they are disease free, which is not always true.

The opposite occurred in a case that I testified for in Syracuse, New York. A patient was sent to the outpatient department of the local hospital for a stress test because of his recent onset of chest pain. This was on a Friday morning. The electrocardiogram portion of the test appeared normal by the cardiologist, and the patient was sent home. The nuclear portion of the study was sent to the chief of pathology, who was in charge of reading nuclear studies. He read the test and interpreted it as positive. He then left the dictation for his secretary to type. Unfortunately, the secretary did not get to the typing until after the weekend. So on Monday, the report was done. In the meantime, the patient thought he was home free and went about his normal exercise program. He died Saturday evening. The patient's primary care physician read the nuclear portion as very positive for heart disease on Monday, but it was then too late. One would ask why the pathologist didn't call the patient or the patient's physician that very day of the test? He answered in court that the hospital had no procedure to deal with this.

Because of my very strong cardiac family history, I personally underwent biannual nuclear stress testing over a ten-year period. Each of the five tests I took was read as normal, with "a little artifact at the inferior portion" of my heart. All five reports stated that this was of no significance. Last year I underwent a stress echo, which showed abnormal wall motion in the corresponding area of the "artifact." A cardiac catheterization (angiogram) proved that I had a singular significant blockage in a major coronary artery. That was significant enough for me.

In Chapter 6 I discussed some patients who had undergone nuclear stress testing with normal results. Despite that, I was compelled to send them for angiography because of the type of pain they were describing.

Oftentimes a relatively young patient will present with chest pains and significant family history (father and brother both had heart attacks), and the patient will be sent for a stress test. When, surprisingly, these otherwise healthy people have positive stress tests, it is obligatory to get a catheterization. Many cardiologists would flinch at that, as they would opt to treat these patients with medication rather than go all the way. My argument is that it is important to know whether these patients really have coronary artery disease or not. Why carry someone the rest of their lives with a label of heart disease when they really may not have it at all? Many young, healthy, muscular men have false-positive stress tests. Or, if they truly do have coronary artery disease, how significant is the disease? Many times the stress test results would suggest mild disease when the catheterization will show horrible multivessel blockage.

Until a few years ago traditional care for coronary artery disease was medication and lifestyle modification (proper diet, exercise, etc.). Then, through the world of cardiac catheterization, angioplasty was introduced. Originally, opening up lesions, partial blockages, by ballooning the blockage and then removing the balloon seemed to work well. Then doctors found that approximately 30 percent of those ballooned lesions closed over and had to be redone.[4]

Then cylindrical tubes (stents) were devised, which were placed in the area that was ballooned and left in place. Raw (untreated) stents had their own inherent problems. One-third of these patients returned when fibrotic (scar) tissue started growing in the area between the stent and the wall of the coronary artery. This scar tissue grew around the stent, causing blockage, emboli, and even myocardial infarctions (heart attacks). By placing a special drug coating on the stents, this scar tissue can be kept to a minimum, especially if the patient takes aspirin and antiplatelet-adhering medications (clopidogrel [Plavix]). This lowers the incidence of clotting and has an almost insignificant number of complications (0.7 percent).[5]

The question of whether to stent or not is one of the most interesting debates in cardiology today. Most studies have shown that patients with stable, nonprogressive cardiac disease, who do not have uncontrollable angina, will not benefit from stenting. Stenting is definitely recommended in acute heart attacks and unstable angina. Immediate mechanical intervention can reverse the heart attack or correct the unstable angina by opening up the clogged coronary artery and will negate the use of multiple cardiac drugs. It is a lifesaving and symptom-relieving procedure. Stable patients can benefit because they would not develop symptoms and would not need medication.

A recent study questioned the benefit of stenting versus bypass surgery. This study was flawed because one-third of the patients developed acute heart attacks during the study and had to undergo catheterization and stenting. The study kept this group in the medication group (which obviously biased the study) and skewed the results. That is, it took one-third of the patients who would have been in the study out of the study, and those were the patients that opted for stenting.[6]

The new controversy in cardiology is how to treat patients who present with acute heart attacks in the local emergency rooms. Up until recently, if the emergency rooms were properly equipped with the thrombolysis medication as well as a cardiologist to administer the medicine, thrombolysis would be the way to go. This works if the patient is treated within the first six hours from the beginning of symptoms. Evidence has now shown that angioplasty and stenting have better outcomes if performed within that same six-hour time frame. This would require immediate transfer to a tertiary care center equipped for cardiac catheterization.

Cardiac catheterization is usually safe in the right hands. One should study the results of heart centers through the various references at the end of this book. Problems can arise with inexperienced "interventionalists." Someone who does one or two procedures a week will probably not be as good as someone who performs ten procedures a day. Some practitioners stent lesions that are not clogged enough (there must be a blockage of 70 to 80 percent to be acceptable for stenting). One of my patients wound up in a distant hospital and was going to have an emergency catheterization for his chest pain. I advised him not to do it and to allow me to transfer him to a major center instead. He elected to undergo the procedure there and was found to have a 50 percent blocked coronary artery. The cardiologist stented the lesion, which was not the cause of the patient's pain. Later, blood tests revealed that the patient had been suffering with an inflammation of the heart.

As I noted earlier, the complication rate of stenting, in good hands, is very low. But the complication rate of not stenting is even lower. Agreeing with your doctor, in principle, which diameter of a lesion should be stented is a good concept to start with. And that is before you ever set foot, or in this case gurney, into the catheterization laboratory.

To recap, coronary artery disease is suspected by symptoms and proven by nuclear or echo stress testing. Using a plain treadmill stress test without nuclear imaging or echo imaging is usually worthless, as the results are only 67 percent accurate.[7] Once someone has a cardiac event (myocardial infarction) or the diagnosis of coronary artery disease, he or she is then placed on various medications.

The practice years ago was to start patients on a class of drugs called beta-blockers. These drugs slow the heart rate and make the heart beat more efficiently. Recent studies suggest that less morbidity (with cerebral vascular accidents as well as heart attacks) and longer mortality can be accomplished with the use of angiotensin-converting enzyme (ACE) inhibitors. This came from results of studies such as the HOPE trial.[8] More recently, the ARIE trial showed similar benefits with ACE inhibitors for patients suffering with acute myocardial infarctions.[9]

The second class of drugs patients are started on are called statins, which lower total values of cholesterol and significantly lower the low-density lipoprotein (LDL) level (this is the bad cholesterol). A very small subset of patients (2 to 5 percent) are evaluated for homocysteine levels.

Years ago it was believed that elevated homocysteine levels were associated with high incidences of coronary artery disease. We started treating these patients with folic acid. What we then learned was that indeed we lowered their homocysteine levels, but these patients were now having an increase—yes, an increase—in heart disease. Folic acid treatment was promptly stopped. As I noted before, only a small subset of familial homocysteinemic patients will have a higher incidence of coronary artery disease. How to identify them and how to treat this disorder, other than lowering cholesterol and using ACE inhibitors, is not really known.[10]

Most recently, cardiac-specific C-reactive protein has become a new investigational tool. It is too early to know whether high levels are associated with a higher incidence of heart disease. What we do know is that taking low-dose aspirin and a statin will lower C-reactive protein levels.[11]

Of course, one's future does not depend on medicine alone, but there must also be a complete lifestyle change. Some of my patients actually accomplish this goal, but for some, unfortunately, it lasts about six to twelve months. Fifty percent of my patients, newly diagnosed with coronary artery disease, make no adjustment whatsoever. I can still smell the cigarette odor, the weight remains elevated, and the muscle mass remains flabby.

In my opinion, many young women worry needlessly about heart disease because their fathers had suffered with premature heart disease or died at a young age because of heart disease. Heart disease mainly affects men, but women are affected by it after menopause. At this point, it affects both genders. This is true unless the mother had heart disease before menopause. If she did, this can then be a hereditable disease for the daughter and therefore concern and caution should abound.

One of the major problems in cardiology is that of pacemakers. One of my patients, Louis, wound up in an emergency room with bradycardia (a very slow heart rate) and symptoms of lightheadedness. The on-call cardiologist insisted on inserting a permanent pacemaker. What was poor, scared Louis to do? When he visited another cardiologist, a week later, it was found that Louis had the slow pulse from some medication he had been taking, and the pacemaker could have been withheld until that medicine cleared his system.

Similar cases occur in patients who have infections (for example, Lyme carditis) and these patients do not need permanent pacemakers, only treatment and observation of their underlying condition. Once a pacemaker is inserted, it becomes part of your heart forever. Insertion of a pacemaker is usually reserved for specific types of heart blockage (complete heart block, second-degree heart block [Mobitz type II], and symptomatic sick sinus syndrome).

Heart disease is managed by frequent stabilization visits to your primary care physician, or a cardiologist, to measure blood pressure, lipid (cholesterol) metabolism, and reactions to medications, as well as electrocardiogram monitoring. When all is stable, the frequency of visits usually falls back to quarterly. Usually, stress testing can then subsequently be performed biannually, unless symptoms dictate otherwise.

Many patients are afraid to take cholesterol-lowering agents because they have heard that liver enzyme abnormalities are a side effect. What they do not realize is that only 5 to 10 percent of patients taking statins get reversible, I stress, *reversible*, liver abnormalities that disappear when the statin is stopped. If they do not take the statin, I argue, you cannot reverse coronary artery disease.

PRESCRIPTION

- If you have a history of heart disease in your family, talk to your doctor about testing and prevention.
- Get a second opinion if you are unsure about your diagnosis.
- Avoid unnecessary procedures if possible; ask your doctor if the procedures are necessary.
- If you are getting a stent, ask your surgeon about his or her experience in placing them.

HOW TO HANDLE THE BIG C
FROM A TO Z: COPING WITH
CANCER TREATMENT

Throughout this book, I stress the fact that the United States is ranked thirty-seventh by the World Health Organization for health care. Nowhere is this more important than in the field of oncology. If we have the right insurance (that costs a lot of money) and if our insurance carriers will pay for the best cancer institutions, then we have the best chance of survival from this dreaded disease. A very close relative was recently diagnosed with mesothelioma. We Googled and researched the top medical centers specializing in this disease and decided that the top choice was in New York and proceeded to make an appointment with one of the world's leading physicians. Wait a minute, we forgot to find out which benefits were offered by his insurance plan. Well, he lives in New Jersey, but his insurance plan did not have coverage for hospitals outside of that state. Of course, if he were hit by a car or had an emergency medical condition, he could go to any hospital, but only in an emergency. After another extensive bout of research, we came up with our second choice, but that center was nowhere as experienced as our first choice. Interestingly, when he first became ill, we kept after his physician's secretary, asking how come she hadn't sent out the referrals necessary for his proper treatment. Well, she said, "I am busy, but the first thing I would tell him is to get a better plan. I would never take that insurance." That was the only plan he was offered by his employer, so it was take it or leave it. Many of our insurance companies have a stock list, or formulary, which limits treatment choices. This is similar to the story at the beginning of this book about how insurance companies make deals with drug companies and try to shy doctors away from prescribing newer, more expensive therapies. Just ask my secretaries who are constantly on the phone asking for permission for the use of a newer medicine.

It is almost like being in a universal health care plan, such as in Canada or Europe, where you get what they offer you. Except there, everyone is covered and everyone is treated the same.

Similar to physicians, hospitals and cancer centers may be certified. Hospitals are certified by the Joint Commission of Hospitals. Checking their Web site, one finds that only 4,000 of the nearly 6,000 hospitals in this country are accredited. According to this site, many of these hospitals (especially in rural areas) have very low ratings.[1] The National Cancer Center, a branch of the National Institutes of Health, certifies major cancer centers (of which, there are only thirty-seven in the United States).[2] This translates into the fact that most cancer patients are treated at their local, community hospital. This may be fine, but one should inquire as to whether the hospital is certified and what level of certification it has been given.

Good nutrition is important to everybody, especially cancer patients. It is evident that everyone needs good nutrition as well as high vitamin levels to get over many diseases. Unfortunately, many people use this argument to promote unproven, uncalled for, nutritional and vitamin alternative therapies. Steve McQueen went to Mexico for coffee enemas to try to cure his liver and colon cancer. He died. A very lovely patient of mine traveled to China to ingest some form of jet fuel for her cancer. She died. People go to all extremes when they hear the word cancer. I met a man, actually a famous baker, who told me that his "wife died of cancer but doctors know the cause and they know the treatment. They are just holding it back from the public."

The U.S. Food and Drug Administration (FDA) labels all vitamin or supplemental products that you buy over the counter "nutritional." Their use by the public carries no liability (unless they are accidently packaged with rat poison). But people buy these supplements because they are being preyed upon. The biggest single company in the supplement market in this country made profits of $200 million last year.[3] The problem is that some patients rush to these alternative routes, expecting miracles, allowing their cancers to worsen, before they ultimately see an oncologist.

The biggest problem with vitamins and supplements, especially antioxidants, is that they may directly inhibit standard treatment and interfere with radiation treatments. Radiation therapy creates free radical oxygen in the cancer cell. Antioxidants inhibit this killing effect. Similarly, antioxidants interfere with the uptake of many cancer medications. So, if you are secretly taking vitamins, please share that information with your oncologist. As a general rule of thumb, you should share information about all prescription and over-the-counter medications that you are taking with your doctor, as well as vitamins and any other supplements. A good doctor will be sure to note this and generate an appropriate course of action.

The Web is a great source of information (as well as misinformation, so be careful). Anytime a patient asks me a question I don't know the answer to, I go on the Web. I once had to chuckle while Googling because it reminded me that when I was growing up, the only way I could get a statistic easily was to check out the almanac. I have included in the resource section at the end of this book many helpful and reliable Web sites. For cancer, you can go to the National Cancer Institute's (NCI) site as well as the American Cancer Society's site. Most cancer centers and hospitals have their own Web sites. As in every field of medicine, it is imperative to become involved and it is imperative to be informed. That is the value of the Web: to give you access to information and treatment alternatives and to find out which treatments may be right for you. I have patients who come in and hand me reams of paper as a result of their research. The information is for you to read and to enable you to talk more equally with your doctor! It will allow you the ability to ask more and intelligent questions. If I haven't heard about it, it probably is some scam. But if I don't know about it, I surely will go to my medical Web sites in a hurry. Often a patient will come in and ask for a special test, one that is only done by some laboratory no one has ever heard of. "But doctor, I read in a magazine that is the only way to diagnose some special disease." Usually the laboratory is either unregistered or the test was never approved by the FDA. Why am I going through this long preamble? Because of our fear of the dreaded "C" word, we will do anything, and often the wrong thing. Our country still houses some of the brightest minds in medicine and their knowledge is there for our benefit. We have to overcome the fear of the illness that we have and take that positive step in intelligently and informatively following our physicians' guidance.

After we have gleaned some knowledge, we now have to check out our surgeons. It can look like a cancer on some test that was given, but a surgeon needs to do a biopsy or to remove the tumor. You should ask for the names of three surgeons who take your insurance. Recently my patient John was found to have cancer on his kidney. Our local urologist is very competent and I would certainly trust him doing that surgery on me if I needed it. John's family insisted that he go to a hospital in New York City, as there, they have the "best" cancer doctors. My urologist would probably not take on a case that is rare or that requires more expertise than he can handle. Similarly, mesothelioma is a tough, difficult tumor to operate on and only top-notch specialists should be doing the surgery. The point that I am trying to make is routine surgery and biopsies can be done locally. Patients who have extensive or rare diseases should be seen at the big centers. John had his surgery and was unhappy because he was far from his home and he found that his home urologist could have easily done the surgery.

When a patient is going to get bad news, it is best to have an advocate along to help. Once patients hear the words "you have cancer" or "you need a heart operation," their systems shut down and they do not hear anything else. Obviously, the calmest person in a fire will find the door. It is important to stay calm and it is important to focus on what is being said. At a time like this your advocate can do the questioning and write down the answers. It is even acceptable to bring a tape recorder so that you can listen to the discussion later or play it when seeking second opinions. Do not be afraid to ask questions, to seek second opinions, and to ask for the range of treatments available for your type of cancer.

One of the best things that has happened lately is the institution of the Navigator Program by the American Cancer Society (ACS). Telephone your local branch of the ACS and talk to them. They can provide an invaluable wealth of impartial and accurate information. They will have many programs to offer you. The program assigns a person to you, who has previously had cancer and whom has undergone your similar scenarios. They are not medical people, but they are trained in how to navigate the system. Many large centers have their own navigator programs that are just as helpful. Various religious organizations have similar programs, stressing knowledge and knowing who the top people for each disease are.

Dealing with cancer must start before the diagnosis is ever made. That sounds strange but in order to find a cancer, you must go to the best places and physicians your pocket, and more importantly, your insurance, can afford.

There are many ways a patient can find out that he or she has cancer. Sometimes it will result from screening tests (mammograms, colonoscopy, prostate screening, etc.). Other times, the diagnosis will result from a consultation with a doctor for a pain syndrome or symptoms that will lead to a biopsy. Often it is found, incidentally, after getting evaluated for a different problem. Many times CT scans are done for abdominal pain, and the bottom portion of the lungs will be visible, revealing a lung lesion.

Many times patients will tell me that they have been recommended, by their friends, to a "specialist" who was tops in the field. Often these recommendations are made because the doctor was nice or had a great personality. Most patients (and nurses included) may never know the medical ability of a particular physician. They have no way of knowing their inadequacies (unless the nurse scrubs with a particular surgeon). A doctor's competency is usually known by his or her peers. Asking doctors who they would have operate on them is a good start. When I want to know who the best breast cancer surgeon is, I ask two or three of my surgical friends. Usually, they will agree on one or two at a great institute. I received my knighthood from the Italian government years ago, because I would translate the medical records from Italy and then find the top physicians in our country who would know how to treat these individuals with rare diseases. Their names are known in the profession and they are published throughout the literature.

Screen testing should be done by a qualified center, and the doctor performing the test should have done many of these tests. It is important to have a mammogram in a center that has high-tech equipment and where it is read by a radiologist who reads hundreds a week and also does biopsies, if needed. The test should be read by two physicians (radiologists), and you should always ask to see the results. Similarly, the biopsy should go out to be read by a lab that specializes in that disease (in this case, breast cancer).

I also what to stress the necessity of proper tissue diagnosis and biopsy of cancer as well as identification errors that occur unfortunately all too often. Some of my patients, under the care of oncologists, who are seemingly in remission, developed another growth or lesion. Mary was doing well and recuperating from her breast cancer (after one year on chemotherapeutic drugs). Unbeknownst to me, her oncologist found a new lung lesion and, assuming this to be a new metastatic lesion in this recently "cured" woman, restarted chemotherapy. Unfortunately, or in this case fortunately, Mary developed a toxic reaction while the oncologist was away and sought my help. The amazing thing is physicians never start chemotherapy unless there has been a tissue diagnosis. Mary never had a biopsy of this new lesion, and when I finally had the pulmonologist do one, it turned out not to be cancer at all. Never accept treatment without a proven biopsy.

Later I discuss the frequency of errors occurring in wrongful identification within laboratories. This happened to one of my patients who was admitted to the hospital after having successful surgery for pancreatic cancer (she had a Whipple procedure). Joan was having postoperative abdominal pain, and a CT scan was performed. What are the odds of another woman of similar age being admitted with the same name but a different oncologist? It is not uncommon for hospitals to have two patients by the same name. The other Joan (Joan 2) was being treated for metastatic colon cancer. She too had a CT scan. Both oncologists did not know the other Joan existed. Joan 2 had a terrible disease, but the hospital reported it out on my patient. So my patient was told by the oncologist that she now had metastatic disease and Joan 2 was told her disease went into remission. This is a true story, and it happens repeatedly, whether the names are the same or not.

If the biopsy is in question (positive, or negative if the lesion looked positive, or equivocal), then it should go out to another lab. Remember, there are labeling mistakes, mistakes in reading, mistakes in telling the wrong person, and delays in telling the right person. Look at the biopsy report and check the names and demographics carefully.

I cannot stress the importance of a second or even a third opinion in reading a biopsy, perhaps even obtaining a superpathology specialist. My colleague was treating a young woman with Hodgkin's disease, which was below the diaphragm and involved her lymph nodes. After the second cycle of therapy, her lymph nodes shrank and she went into remission. After the fifth cycle she started to become short of breath and her lung x-ray revealed pulmonary infiltrates. He thought his patient may be having infiltrates secondary to the chemotherapy drugs, as this is a common side effect. The prospect of Hodgkin's recurring so soon after remission was considered, but my friend found that rather odd, especially since the recurrence occurred in a new place, the lungs. A biopsy was performed at the local hospital and it was read as positive for Hodgkin's. A reflex biopsy (a second slide is sent to another lab for confirmation) was then sent to a tertiary hospital, as is the custom. Again, this was read as positive. At this point, the pathology specimens were indicating to treat the Hodgkin's.

Because it clinically did not make sense, a superspecialist pathologist in Hodgkin's and lung disease was found and the slides were sent to her. The diagnosis was an unrelated new pulmonary disease (bronchiolitis obliterans). This disease causes scarring of the lungs and if the patient would have been treated with chemotherapy, her lungs would have gotten worse.

The approach to cancer therapy depends on the treating physician and the institution where he or she practices. Some oncologists are extremely aggressive, while others may take a more standard approach. Some even opt for a mild reduced approach to minimize the toxic effects of many of these medications. Most important, you have to inform yourself on all of the therapy modalities available. These can be found on the National Cancer Center's Web site, as well as other cancer Web sites listed in the resources section of this book.

Most often, there should be no rushing into therapy. One's cancer took a long time to grow and waiting a few weeks usually does not matter, though there are exceptions to this rule, so do consult closely with your doctor about your particular situation. Before jumping into an irreversible program, you should be well informed and you need to discuss your treatment with one or two physicians.

Cancer therapy is usually initiated after staging. This basically refers to how much cancer volume a patient has. The more the cancer, the higher the stage! Stage 1 is confined to one organ and one area/one lump that is small. These are almost always treated with surgery to remove the disease and may, occasionally, be followed by radiation and/or chemotherapy (if it was a very aggressive cancer). Stage 2 cancers are either bigger lumps (more than an inch or two) or those that have spread to nearby lymph nodes. Lymph nodes are the drainage system of the body's waste. This stage is also treated with surgery, but more often followed by radiation and chemotherapy (as the relapse rates start to rise in stage 2). Stage 3 disease is advanced, usually locally. The treatment is usually preoperative radiation and/or chemotherapy, followed by surgery (providing the initial treatment worked). Stage 4 cancer is advanced and spread to other sites of the body. Treatments are usually medical, meaning chemotherapies and other drugs. Stages 1 and 2 cancers are usually curable, while stages 3 and 4 are often more difficult and sometimes have serious outcomes, but there are people who survive and even thrive after advanced stages of cancer.

Chemotherapeutic agents are known for their toxicities, and I am sure that many patients die from the treatment instead of the disease. All of these side effects must be explained to you. Of special concern is the infiltration of chemotherapeutic agents into the deep skin (this occurs if the needle comes out of the vein while still in the arm). Deep tissue burns are horrible complications that have dying people suffering even more. Physicians push for permanent intravenous devices (port lines) to be inserted to avoid this complication. A small percentage of these ports may become infected, especially if they are in for a year or longer. Some may cause thrombosis (blockage of a vein) with pain and swelling. But in my observation, these complications occur much less than deep tissue burns.

Cancer therapy has become a big business. Hospitals are building outpatient cancer centers and going into direct competition with local oncologists. Rather than losing lots of money to keep patients hospitalized, much more money can be made if the patient is treated at these outpatient facilities. Years ago oncologists made large sums of money by "selling" the cancer drugs to the patient and administering the agent intravenously. The insurance industry has cut back payments for these profits on the chemical agents, but do pay $130 per hour, for up to two hours, to administer the drug intravenously. This figure is taken right from the Medicare code books. When to stop chemotherapy brings up some interesting facts. The National Cancer Society has guidelines, but these are only guidelines and they do not take into account the nuances of the disease. Some patients want to keep on therapy longer than their cure, as a safety net. Are doctors continuing the therapy for monetary gain?

The job of oncologists is one of providing patients with all of their options, as well as the statistical chances of survival. Their job is not to railroad patients into one treatment or another, but to guide patients through the maze of varied therapies. This should include experimental treatments that are available for certain aggressive tumors.

Alternative treatments to standard cancer therapy are classified into two categories: those that are trying to treat the cancer and those that are adjunctive (helping the patient while on therapy). Adjunctive therapies have been found to be very helpful. Aroma therapy, deep muscle massage, and healing hands can all be calming and help patients get through these really hard times. Patients should also be sent for psychological counseling as well as nutritional counseling. Organizations such as the American Cancer Society and Gilda's Club have multiple support groups, both for patients as well as their families. When cancer strikes, it affects everyone in the family. All become survivors! Gilda's Club has a great program to help children understand and deal with family members who have cancer. Acupuncture as well as music therapy can be helpful in controlling pain. Talk therapy is very important because it keeps the disease out in the forefront and not hidden. Sharing with others has certainly helped many patients deal and cope.

Alternative therapies that seek to directly treat cancer are dangerous and should be avoided. They will not be covered by any insurance carrier (for good reasons) and are usually quite expensive, easily draining your resources. Just remember the results of Steve McQueen's coffee enemas!

There are many different types of cancer, and doctors do not always have the answers. But developing a relationship with an oncologist and his or her team can help head off any unintended errors. Keeping informed, taking care of your overall health, and following through with treatment can combine to help you survive. Fighting cancer is always difficult, no matter what stage or level of trouble you find yourself in. Therefore, the more information you have to make the tough decisions, the better off you will be.

PRESCRIPTION

- How do you beat the odds? Get your annual physical, Pap test, mammogram, x-ray, etc. If there is a strong family history of colon cancer, then you need a colonoscopy every five years, starting around age 45. If not, then colonoscopies are suggested every seven to ten years, starting at age 50.
- Do not ignore signs of disease. I have a relative that had rectal bleeding for one year before he had the courage to see a doctor. He now wears a colostomy bag.
- Do regular self breast and genital examinations. Consider that any changes (lumps, etc.) are abnormal until proven otherwise.
- If there is a new lesion in your body, you need a biopsy.
- Double read on biopsies or x-rays is your new mantra.
- Most cancers are curable if they are caught early.
- You cannot fight your genes, however. To forestall most diseases you must have a good lifestyle, exercise, eat healthfully, not smoke, or not do harmful things in excess.

9

BABY BOOM OR BUST: HOW TO STROLL THROUGH MATERNITY, NEONATAL, AND FERTILITY ISSUES

The journey into womanhood starts with a visit to a gynecologist. When to start these visits varies from doctor to doctor. Some suggest that a young woman should see one between the ages of 13 to 15. A woman should definitely start visiting the gynecologist each year if she has been sexually active (and age does not count). If she is not sexually active, the recommended age varies, so if you are a parent and have a teenage daughter, talk to your gynecologist to get a recommended age for your child's first visit. The American College of Obstetricians and Gynecologists recommends that Pap smears be done annually, by age 21, or within three years of first sexual intercourse. A woman should, however, always visit the gynecologist if she experiences bleeding after sexual intercourse, bleeding between periods, or has any persistent or unusual vaginal discharge. Postmenopausal women who bleed should run, not walk, to their gynecologist at the first sign of bleeding. With the annual Pap smear, all women should have a pelvic examination (checking for abnormalities or infections). Many women may have a disease without knowing of it, as many sexually transmitted diseases (STDs) may not have symptoms early in their course. Furthermore, ovarian cysts, uterine fibroids, endometriosis, and even cancer may be found during these visits. Irregular menses and ovarian cysts can be easily treated with birth control pills.

Many women suffer anxiety when it is time for their yearly vaginal examinations. To mitigate this anxiety, a patient can first determine if having a male or female doctor would make this more comfortable. A female nurse or assistant is usually present during these examinations, no matter the gender of the doctor, both for the protection of the patient as well as the physician. Sometimes in an office setting with mixed groups of gynecologists you can try one, then the next year, the other.

During your annual examination, your blood pressure, vital signs, and weight should be taken. Some gynecologists like to be your PCP. However, sometimes they are not that well trained for cardiac, pulmonary, or other internal medicine fields to act as your sole PCP. My gynecologist friends may take offense at this, but I have trained for years in those subspecialties and they have not. When I presented this thought to my obstetrics/gynecology friend, he said, "No offense is taken, as long as you didn't do Pap tests." An annual visit for a "female" examination and symptomatic visits during the year would be just fine. During this annual visit you should also be given a thorough breast examination accompanied by a lesson in self-examination. Doctors check your breasts for any changes in the skin (dimpling or redness) as well as for lumps and nipple discharge. Axillary and supraclavicular (above the clavicles) lymph nodes are checked for enlargement.

While performing a Pap smear, the physician could also be taking smears for STDs and genital warts (human papillomavirus [HPV]). If it is your first examination, you will note that the doctor uses latex gloves, with a lubricant, so as not to hurt you. If you are aware that you have an allergy to latex, be sure you let the doctor know. During the Pap test, named after Dr. George Papanicolaou, the doctor takes a cell sample from the cervix for examination.

There has recently arisen a large controversy regarding annual Pap testing. There have been recommendations by various medical organizations suggesting that Pap smears be done every three years, after two or three consecutive Paps have been normal. It appears this is primarily driven by attempts to reduce the costs of medical care. Although not incorrect regarding the lower risk of abnormal Paps in those groups of women, it carries significant danger.[1] For one, it took physicians decades to persuade women to have regular preventive gynecological visits. It finally became a standard procedure that most women follow. But if they are told that they do not need a Pap, they simply won't go to their gynecologist. In public perception, a Pap smear is synonymous with a gynecological visit. No Pap smear, no visit. Patients will skip a year or even two, possibly risking their health as a potential health issue can arise during "off" years. Deciding how often to have a Pap should be something you discuss with your gynecolo-

gist and should depend on your history, age, sexual activity, and other factors. There are many women who have had "bad" Pap tests less than three
years after their first intercourse.[2] In addition, pathology reports can be
erroneous, so always double check with your doctor before assuming a test
is accurate. Many gynecologists will call only with an abnormal result, but
because doctors are busy and can sometimes overlook reports, it would be
a good idea to call anyway to get results, just to be sure.

Another controversy is that of specifically testing for HPV and vaccination for prevention of certain types of HPV. The genital human papillomavirus, a virus commonly transmitted sexually, can turn some normal
cells of the cervix into abnormal ones. This can possibly lead to precervical
or cervical cancer. There are about forty types of HPV that can infect the
genitals of men and women. It is so common that most people are infected
at some time in their lives. Some HPV types can cause genital warts, while
other types can cause cellular changes that rarely lead to cervical cancer. It
is not known why, but most of the time, the HPV goes away by itself (usually within two years) and causes no health problems at all. Most people
who contract HPV do so when they first start to have sexual intercourse.

A Pap smear is taken to check for abnormal cells that rarely can turn into
cervical cancer. Getting regular Pap smears is the best way to prevent cervical cancer. Most cases of abnormal Pap tests (or those that are inconclusive)
turn out not to be cervical cancer. If a Pap test is negative, it is usually not
necessary to do a test for HPV since most women have the virus and most
will cure themselves. If a Pap test comes back positive, it is at this point an
HPV test can be helpful. The company that developed the HPV test spent a
lot of money for development and getting it approved. They want to recoup
the investment and make a profit: all well and good. But unless you really
need the test, you may decide to opt not to have it. Consulting with your
doctor about the need for this test is always a good idea.

Most competent gynecologists request their cytology labs to perform so-
called reflex HPV. What this means is that normal, complete Pap tests are
just that and need no further testing.[3] Checking for and finding a positive
HPV on the smear will not change the diagnosis of a normal Pap. It will,
however, upset a great number of affected young women without offering
them any solution. The psychological impact can be considerable. On the
other hand, the finding of an abnormal Pap (mild dysplasia, etc.) has to be
further evaluated properly and it is safe to assume that HPV is there.[4]

The Pap test is just a screening test. As such, it has to be easy, reproduc-
ible, fairly specific, and sensitive (and cheap). It is, however, not diagnostic.

If it comes back abnormal, your doctor will need to move to the next level: colposcopy. Colposcopy literally means looking into the vagina. This is done with a binocular microscope, looking for microscopic abnormalities (and of course, doing a biopsy of them). Oftentimes the results may come back as cervical dysplasia. This is a condition that spans the very broad spectrum of changes from normal tissue to real cervical cancer. Dysplasia turns up and scares so many women, and yet it is not cancer and may be secondary to a variety of things from inflammation to infection or a fungus. I get perhaps one call a month from a patient who has been told that their gynecologist found dysplasia and they want to know what they should do next. Getting a second opinion is always a good idea, and discussing outcomes and any necessary treatments for anything your doctor does find is advisable.

MAMMOGRAMS

Women with normal family histories usually have a baseline mammogram at age 37. It is then followed from age 40 to 50 with mammograms biannually. At age 50, they are done annually. Younger women do not typically have mammograms because the texture of the breast tissue is difficult to evaluate for cancer. On the other hand, breast cancer in older women first may show as microcalcifications before they are palpable. However, no matter your age, if you find a lump, have it checked out as soon as you can. Lumps may or may not show up on a mammogram and must be seen by a breast specialist. Women with strong family histories of breast cancer should have their mammograms annually. We offer these women breast cancer markers (found in blood testing) as well as chromosomal studies. (Chapter 14 gives a deeper look into the pitfalls of mammography.) Most baseline mammograms come with a report suggesting a follow-up visit. Many times these are just to track any changes in the breast tissue to rule out abnormalities. Again, do not wait to hear from your doctor assuming results are normal. Call and ask to hear the results and get a written report.

INFERTILITY

Experts in infertility are called reproductive endocrinologists. They consider a couple to be infertile if:

1. The female is unable to carry a pregnancy to full term.
2. If, after being contraceptive free for twelve months, the couple has not conceived (if the woman is less than 35 years old) or if over 35, the couple has not conceived, after six months.

Most couples who have regular sex will conceive within a year. However, one out of seven couples will have difficulty. There are many causes for infertility, which are evaluated by "fertility specialists." Interestingly, the reason is unknown in 25 percent of these couples. However, it is a fifty-fifty diagnosis of male-factor versus female-factor infertility.

The first step is for the male to obtain a sperm evaluation. This will reveal if sperm are present and if they function properly. I once had a patient who was trying to conceive with her husband (who had been married previously). After two years, they were sent to a fertility specialist, who after careful questioning, realized that the male had previously had a vasectomy and never told his new bride. One would be surprised how many women take birth control pills, not realizing that this will interfere with conception. If there is a problem with sperm, the male is checked for endocrine disorders as well as for a varicocele (an abnormally large network of veins in the scrotum, which is otherwise innocuous). A certain percentage of varicoceles can cause infertility, which, when removed, will allow fertilization.

Then, if the male is normal, the women's reproductive organs are evaluated for abnormalities, scarring from previous surgery or infection, and patent fallopian tubes.

If all else fails, couples can elect assisted reproductive technologies (ART). One form is artificial insemination, where sperm (either from the mate or, if infertile, from a catalog of registered donors). There are a range of technologies, so if you find yourself having difficulty conceiving or carrying a baby to term, discuss other options with your doctor.

Some couples elect in vitro fertilization (IVF) without fear of becoming the "Octomom." This phenomenon is extremely rare and could have been avoided had the doctor involved not transferred multiple embryos or had the mother opted for a selective reduction of the implanted embryos. Any woman undergoing IVF can recall the painful injections and carefully monitored hormonal levels with daily blood testing. If you opt to elect IVF as a treatment, check to see that it is your name on the tube. Stories of mixups often make headlines, and you probably do not want to be a victim of such a mixup.

Some alternative or complements to assisted reproductive technologies include acupuncture, group psychological intervention, and manual manipulative physical therapy.

IVF is very expensive for both the fertility specialist and the patient as the medication and frequent ultrasound examinations are costly and time-consuming. Many insurance companies may not offer adequate coverage, and many women go abroad to countries where the costs are a third to a quarter less than they are in the United States. Yes, I said a third to a quarter of what they are here! However, not all couples will be able to conceive with the assistance of these technologies. Some may opt to adopt or to hire a gestational carrier (surrogate) to bear their biological child. In these instances, a good infertility practice will be able to set you up with legal advisors to arrange such a situation. Don't leave yourself open to legal complications by not seeking legal advice in such instances.

CONCEPTION AND PREGNANCY

As the slogan is often quoted, the educated consumer makes the best customer. When approaching pregnancy, labor, delivery, and the postpartum period, one should become deeply informed. So much will happen to the woman's body (the least of which can be varicose veins and hemorrhoids), as well as to interpersonal relationships (between husband and wife).

Prenatal care will involve a careful history of your illnesses as well as possible genetic familial defects that may affect your child. Blood tests are ordered for blood typing as well as the Rh factor, which can cause problems with the fetus. Blood testing is also done for STDs, including HIV. Cervical smears are done similarly for STDs as well as for strep group B, which is an infection that can affect the newborn.

It would be impossible to cover every possible thing that could go wrong in a pregnancy in this book, and the truth is that the vast majority of pregnancies result in the birth of a healthy child. That does not mean something cannot go wrong, and it does not mean that if something does go wrong it cannot be addressed prior to birth. Your first line of defense should be educating yourself and getting consistent, and good, prenatal care for yourself and your baby from the start. Throughout a pregnancy, obstetricians rely on frequent ultrasound examinations of the pelvis and fetus. Some doctors will evaluate kick counts (the amount of kicking done by the baby). A healthy baby kicks the same amount each day. Then there is the electronic fetal monitoring, which will help detect developing problems the baby may have later in the pregnancy. Alphafetoprotein testing (AFP) is a screening test using maternal blood to test for abnormalities in the growing fetus. It was found to be an imperfect tool by many obstetricians (even the quadruple screen). It was reported in mathematical odds and at best was quite confusing, because there was always some risk involved. Many obstetricians now use the new first trimester screen (ultrascreen), which involves sonographic measurement of the thickness of the baby's neck and two blood tests (PAPP-A and free beta HCG). It is performed twelve to fourteen weeks into a pregnancy and seems very solid in picking up trisomies 21, 13, and 18. The early detection of these major birth defects is important to many pregnant women.

Various blood and perhaps amniotic fluid analyses can determine whether the baby is affected with cystic fibrosis, Down syndrome, or other disorders. Further testing, such as chorionic villus sampling (CVS), is done for various trisomies and neural tube defects. Many of these tests can provide a false positive, or false negative, and may have to be repeated. Most amniocentesis tests, where a sample of the amniotic fluid is taken and analyzed for genetic abnormalities, are more accurate, although they do carry a 1 percent miscarriage rate. You should inform your doctor when you first suspect you are pregnant, and on your first visit go over the various testing that he or she offers and when those tests should be conducted. On the bright side, most babies are born healthy and disease free.

During this prenatal period, it is important to take a prenatal vitamin fortified with iron and folic acid. The iron helps counteract anemia, which can very often arise, and the folic acid is associated with reduced neural tube defects. One should also take calcium to build the baby's bones and teeth. The doctor will also recommend a diet high in protein, the body's "building block." This helps build the baby's muscles and tissues.

Weight gain has always been a thorny problem. Many women put on too much weight and have trouble taking it off for the rest of their lives. Years ago, many obstetricians did not bother reminding women about their excessive weight gain, because, aside from some rare complications, it did not matter. However, women should realize that careful monitoring of their weight is important, if only for the reason they may be stuck with it the rest of their lives. Maintaining a healthy weight, eating right, and getting exercise will help prevent weight-related problems. Most doctors, however, recommend not starting a new course of exercise while pregnant, suggesting instead to stick with what your body is used to. If you are a smoker, it is time to quit, as it can lead to low birth weight babies, and it can put the baby at risk for asthma and sudden infant death syndrome (SIDS). If you drink, it is also time to quit, although some doctors feel that a drink every now and then does not seem to be a problem, as no one knows exactly how much alcohol it takes to harm the fetus. Others advise total abstinence. High amounts of alcohol consumption often lead to fetal alcohol syndrome, which may lead to joint and limb defects, mental retardation, as well as heart defects.

One of the most common complaints of a pregnant woman (which is a redundant statement as men don't get pregnant) is backache. Women assume funny postures to offset the extra weight gain. Furthermore, the extra weight gain puts strain on the back. Exercising to strengthen and stretch the back muscles should help alleviate back pain. Other possible bodily changes include varicose veins, swelling of the vulva, hemorrhoids, bleeding gums, and other minor ailments. Discuss these with your doctor if you should experience any of them.

The early signs of pregnancy, swelling of the breasts, nausea, and increased urination (due to the increase of hormones), gradually disappear after the first trimester. Some may suffer with nausea and vomiting into the third month (nausea gravidarum). Some women go on to suffering with heartburn throughout their pregnancy. The increased hormones cause the esophageal valve to stay relaxed and open, causing reflux.

Lastly, emotions are rapidly changing and depression is one symptom that has to be carefully monitored, especially if there was a prenatal history. If you begin to feel depressed or have sudden severe mood swings, discuss these with your doctor or with a licensed therapist. Now is not the time to conceal how you are feeling, and a doctor can more readily help you if he or she knows what is happening.

There are various methods of birth delivery. There is one method involving hypnotism (hypno birth). Another, proposed by a Russian, Igor Tjarkovsky, and improved by French physician Michel Ordent, became popular in the 1980s in the United States. In this method a woman is placed in a tub during labor and the baby is born under water. The Bradley method strongly encourages the birthing woman to not take any drug at all during delivery. I am a traditionalist. When the pain becomes unbearable, it is time for an epidural!

The decision to have a Cesarean (known as C sections) delivery depends on either a medical emergency or the desire to have a planned delivery. C sections occur in 25 percent of deliveries. As I will discuss a little later, many obstetricians opt for C section deliveries to avoid being sued for intrauterine fetal brain damage. Before opting for a C section, discuss all of the options with your doctor and be sure you are aware of the complications and the added recovery time. Vaginal delivery can also pose risks, and these too should be discussed with your doctor in advance to minimize any complications. Going into the process with an arsenal of information may help mitigate any feelings of anxiety associated with delivering a baby. Asking about your doctor's background and experience in all kinds of deliveries is reasonable, and if your doctor balks at such questions, it may be time to find a new doctor.

Of all the postpartum changes, and unfortunately there will be lots of changes, the most worrisome is depression. About 10 percent of new mothers will suffer from postpartum depression. This occurs more frequently in women who have suffered with depression in the past. One's family has to be put on notice, as careful observation is necessary. I had a patient who suffered with postpartum depression after her pregnancies and tried to commit suicide after each one, a few weeks to months after delivery. She always chose the middle of the night. On the last attempt, I asked if she ever considered trying the attempt during the day so that I could sleep through the night! I had to go to the emergency room on each attempt. She laughed at my humor, but it was really kidding "on the square." If you suspect you are experiencing postpartum depression, get help immediately. Do not let a doctor or any other person dismiss your concerns. Postpartum depression is real, and it needs to be treated.

CONTROVERSIES IN OBSTETRICS/GENECOLOGY

Gardasil is a recent vaccination developed to be administered to teenage girls to prevent some of the HPV types associated with changes of cervical cells and hence prevent many cases of cervical cancer. Forty years ago, the government spent a million dollars on a campaign to encourage everyone to get the "million dollar rubella umbrella." Even though the vaccine had not yet proven effective (it was later found that the protection wore off in 20 percent of those who received it), everyone had to have it. A similar

thing happened with the chickenpox vaccine. Many adults who received
the chickenpox vaccination as children are now susceptible to coming
down with varicella (chickenpox), since its protection also decreases over
time. In fact, a local young gynecologist got deathly ill with chickenpox last
year. Childhood diseases that occur in adults can be deadly. So, with that in
mind, there is some resentment that this misrepresented "cancer vaccine,"
Gardasil, came on the market, seemingly fast tracked through the FDA. It
was accompanied with political pressures and advertised with much more
than a million dollar umbrella.[5] Cervical cancer deaths numbered just under 3,900 cases in the United States in 2005.[6] From 1996 to 2005 there was
a significant yearly decrease in the rates of new cervical cancer incidences
and the Centers for Disease Control felt that these trends suggested a
continued decrease overall.[7] According to an NIH report, the incidence is
decreasing by 5 percent yearly because of better awareness and increased
Pap testing (and not because of Gardasil).[8]

The *New England Journal of Medicine* published an editorial, which was
reported in the May 14, 2007, issue of *Woman's Health/Gynecology News*,
that described over 1,600 adverse reactions to Gardasil. A report in the *Los
Angeles Times* in 2008 showed that there were thirty-one cases of Guil-
lain-Barré syndrome and over fifteen deaths associated with the vaccine.
It does not seem like a public help to me, especially if millions of young
women are encouraged to have the vaccination. To further complicate the
matter, the vaccine will not work if the woman has already been exposed
to HPV. As recently as August 2008, the *New England Journal of Medicine*
cautioned about HPV vaccine use.[9] Most cases of cervical cancers can be
detected early on with proper Pap testing and most are treatable.

HORMONE REPLACEMENT THERAPY

Another controversy is that of the use of hormone replacement therapy
(HRT). Superficially looking at the topic, why wouldn't a woman go on
HRT? Hot flashes, night sweats, sleep disorders, depression, osteoporosis,
dry irritated vagina, and a host of other problems are no fun at all. The
thought of growing a beard and getting stretched, flabby skin is another
motivation. But of course, there are drawbacks that have to be carefully
examined. One has to look into one's family history for cancer (especially
of the female organs), as well as a history of clotting disorders.

HRT was carefully studied in a series of trials called the Women's Health Initiative and showed that there is a small increase in the rate of breast cancer (in those women taking a combination of progesterone and estrogen). The study also showed an increased rate of ovarian cancer, heart disease, and blood clotting. The incidence of these diseases starts its increase in women who are ten years or more past the start of menopause.[10]

However, by use of the above combination, one can be protected from endometrial cancer and possibly from colon cancer. So there is medical evidence for and against HRT. If one had a history of deep vein thrombosis or pulmonary embolization, or if one had a personal history of endometrial, breast, or ovarian cancer, I, personally, would strongly recommend not taking the chance.

BIRTH DEFECTS

One of the most controversial causes for litigation in the field of obstetrics is that of whether neonatal encephalitis and cerebral palsy are caused from medical malpractice. On January 31, 2003, a joint announcement was made by the American College of Obstetrics and Gynecology (ACOG) and the American Academy of Pediatrics (AAP) on their long-term study of newborn brain injuries. The conclusion was that less than 10 percent of cases of neurologic impairment in newborns are the result of events occurring in labor, and, of these, the majority were not preventable. The report revealed that the vast majority of these diseases originate from developmental or metabolic abnormalities, autoimmune and coagulation defects, infection, trauma, or combinations of these factors. It also revealed that many obstetricians pushed quickly for Cesarean sections at the first sign of any fetal distress (by fetal heart rate monitor), so as to limit the possibility of hypoxia (slowing of oxygen supply to the brain) during childbirth.[11]

Another news release by ACOG, on November 3, 2006, revealed that in a survey 70 percent of obstetricians/gynecologists have made changes to their practices because of the lack of available or affordable medical liability insurance, and 65 percent have made changes because of the risk or fear of liability claims or litigation. Eight percent have stopped practicing obstetrics altogether, suggesting that women's access to health care may be hurt by the liability crisis.[12] Certainly, malformations and malpractice occur in every field, including that of obstetrics, brachial plexus deformities being one of many. The obstetricians' objection, according to my colleagues, is that they are sued for every poor outcome; using brain injuries as the prime example, when 90 percent are proven to be formed in utero, long before childbirth.

Many birth defects are congenital, others can be caused by injury, still others have no known underlying cause. The best way to guard against birth defects and injury is to educate yourself, get good prenatal care, and choose an obstetrician/gynecologist with experience and a good track record. If you feel uncomfortable with your obstetrician for any reason, try to find another with whom you feel more comfortable. Research the hospital where you will deliver your baby, and if you have a choice of hospitals, choose one where they are equipped to handle emergencies, either with you or with the baby. Do not be afraid to ask questions, and seek a second opinion if you are given a difficult diagnosis.

PRESCRIPTION

- Call your doctor when you get your first positive pregnancy test and set up an appointment.
- Follow your doctor's advice about weight gain, exercise, and vitamins.
- Be sure to ask about the purpose and timing of all testing during pregnancy.
- Research the hospital where you will deliver. Is there a neonatal intensive care unit as well as a neonatologist should something go wrong during the delivery?
- If you are a high-risk pregnancy (your age factor, multiple pregnancy, chronic illness), you should be followed by a "high-risk" specialist.
- Discuss medications (many are related to fetal injury).
- If undergoing IVF, be sure to check labels before, during, and after specimens are given, cultured, and returned.
- Any abnormal test (Pap, blood, etc.) should be repeated. Errors occur hundreds of times daily at your local hospital.

10

YOU GIVE ME FEVER: INFECTION AND COMMUNICABLE DISEASES

> The ideal way to get rid of any infectious disease would be to shoot instantly any person who comes down with it.
>
> —Henry Louis Mencken[1]

Infectious diseases are probably the most common reason for patients to seek help from their physicians or from the emergency room. In general, there are two types of infection: local and systemic. Years ago we used to teach medical students the Latin phrase *Rubor, Calor, Tumor, Dolor*, and *Functio Laesa*. Redness, warmth, swelling, pain, and loss of function classically describe a local infection. These infections occur when there is a break in the skin barrier (cuts or bruises), allowing bacteria into a wound. In the case of surgical wound infections, either the surgical site was not adequately cleansed or the surgeon (or nurse or other technician) accidently introduced bacteria into the wound (cough, sneeze, gloves not cleaned). Infected surgical wounds almost always occur at the moment of surgery.

One of the saddest examples of an infection getting into a wound at the time of the procedure was in a case I testified for against an emergency room physician. The doctor suspected meningitis in an ill infant. A spinal tap was performed, which turned out to be completely normal. Unfortunately, the child was brought back to the emergency room six hours later with true signs and symptoms of full-blown meningitis. The child did not survive the illness. The offending organism was found to be *Staphylococcus*, which is the predominant organism on that portion of one's back (where the spinal tap is performed). Obviously, the skin was not adequately sterilized or the hands of the physician were contaminated.

Many patients have gotten cortisone injections in their joints by orthopedists or their primary care physicians. Joint space infections can similarly occur if the site is not adequately sterilized. As an expert in infectious diseases, I have treated many of these "physician-induced" infections. Jane, a neighbor and patient, was given a cortisone injection in her foot for severe pain and swelling from her underlying rheumatoid arthritis. She soon developed a serious infection, involving the bones of her foot. Because she lives in the country, she often walks her property in bare feet, and her feet were colonized with an unusual bacterium, avian mycobacteria, which her specialists never cultured for. This delayed the diagnosis and treatment of her osteomyelitis (bone infection), resulting in surgical removal of part of her foot.

Systemic infections imply that circulating organisms (bacterial, viral, or fungal) are in our bloodstream or organ systems. Signs of fever, chills, aches, confusion, fatigue, or shaking usually accompany systemic infections.

Certain bacteria, known for that area or organ, colonize many of our organ systems. Our skin is a "barrier organ" that is known to be normally colonized by *Staphylococci*. The skin around the anus will have Gram-negative organisms from the colon. Toes may have fungus or may have unusual bacteria, especially if that person walks barefoot.

The upper respiratory tree has lots of harmless *Streptococci*, *Staphylococci*, and some Gram-negative organisms. Knowing where the infection started will usually be a great clue as to which bacteria are causing the infection. Thus treatment can be started intelligently, while cultures take their time growing in the laboratory.

All systemic infections, whether they are due to bacteria or viruses, *must* be diagnosed and treated as an urgent matter. Any delay in treatment may lead to an unfavorable result. One of the most valuable signs indicating infection is fever. Easily defined, fever is the elevation of body temperature above the normal level, which in humans is 98 degrees Fahrenheit (37°C), when measured orally. This number was obtained by measuring the temperatures of thousands of people and then taking an average. It is considered to be a symptom of a disorder, rather than a disease in itself. Under normal conditions, the heat that is generated by the burning of food by the body (that is calories) is dissipated through such processes as perspiration and breathing. It is believed that infectious diseases, injury to the body tissues, and other conditions that cause inflammation lead to the release of prostaglandins (a type of hormone), which bind to sites in the hypothalamus (the center of temperature control in the body). The rise in temperature that is triggered as a result acts as part of the body's defense against infection. These reactions to fever increase the activity of white blood cells and diminish the ability of the invading bacteria to thrive. Fever can cause the body to feel weak, exhausted, and sometimes depleted of body fluids (through excessive perspiration). High fevers may even cause convulsions. In years past and before the days of antibiotics, heavy metals (such as mercury and arsenic) were found to induce very high fevers and were subsequently used to treat diseases such as syphilis. The bacteria causing these infections could not live under these high temperatures and would die. (This was depicted in the movie *Out of Africa*.) In medical parlance, we use the word pyrexia (Greek *pyretos*: fire) or a febrile response (Latin: *febris* or fever). The person who is developing a fever has a cold sensation and an increase in heart rate, muscle tone, and shivering attempt.

Patterns of a fever can often suggest the underlying cause:

- Severe shaking chills: usually connote bacteria being released into the bloodstream (bacterial sepsis) from such places as a urinary tract infection or pneumonia, for example. One to two hours later, the patient will develop a high fever.
- Continuous fevers: where the temperature remains above normal throughout the whole day and does not fluctuate more than 1 degree Celsius during that twenty-four-hour period. This suggests urinary tract infections, lobar pneumonia, brucellosis, typhus, or typhoid fever.
- Intermittent fevers: elevated temperatures are present for only some hours of the day and become normal for remaining hours (kala azar, pyemia, septicemia, or malaria). Malaria is a parasitic infection that can be caused by a few types of parasites. Each one of these parasites causes different types of fever patterns. Amazingly, Hippocrates was able to measure these patterns, almost two thousand years ago, before the invention of a thermometer. These malarial fevers occur in a twenty-four-hour fever period (quotidian), a forty-eight-hour period (tertian fever), and a seventy-two-hour period (quartan fever). That is, the fever lasts, in the latter example, for seventy-two hours and then goes away for a few days. This is important because we know that one parasite, *Plasmodium malariae*, is the cause of the seventy-two-hour fever and therefore we know which antimalarial medicine specifically to use.

- Remittent fever: the temperature remains above normal throughout the day and fluctuates more than 1 degree Celsius in twenty-four hours. Infective endocarditis is an infection with a remittent pattern.
- Fevers that occur within a half hour of taking a medication can often suggest the medication as the source of the temperature elevation.
- Intermittent high spiking fevers, preceded by severe shaking chills, often suggest a blocked tube or duct. This is seen in patients with gallbladders or urinary tracts blocked by a stone.
- Fevers with stepwise decreases, that is staying on a plateau for a few days and then decreasing to a lower plateau for a few days, indicate gradual healing, especially if the patient is on an antibiotic.

Fever is defined as a rectal temperature or otic temperature (via the ear) at or over 100.4°F (38°C). This is equivalent to an oral temperature at or over 99.5°F (37.5°C). If you do not own a thermometer, you can take a pulse. The pulse will be ten points higher for every degree rise in temperature. If you know that your normal pulse is seventy and while you are ill it is ninety, then your temperature will be two degrees higher than normal. In this case, instead of the normal temperature of 98.6°F, the fever would be 100.6°F.

CAUSES OF FEVER

There are several causes of fever:

- Fevers can be directly caused by a drug (progesterone or perhaps chemotherapeutic agents, which cause tumor necrosis) or as an adverse reaction to a drug (allergic reaction to penicillin or a sulfa drug). Some drugs cause fever after they are withdrawn (heroin or fentanyl).
- Cancers (most commonly renal cancer, leukemia, and lymphoma)
- Infectious agents (the common cold, influenza, malaria, infectious mononucleosis, HIV)
- Various skin inflammations (boils, abscess)
- Immunological diseases (collagen diseases: lupus erythematosus, sarcoidosis, rheumatoid arthritis, as well as inflammations of the intestine; colitis or Crohn's disease)
- Metabolic disorders (porphyria or gout)

- Poor inflation of the lungs (atelectasis), such as after chest or abdominal surgery
- Thromboembolic processes (pulmonary embolism or deep vein thrombosis)

With all of the above considered, a physician should approach a febrile patient in the following manner. The patterns should be studied carefully. If the fever came on gradually, this would suggest a viral infection. Did it occur abruptly, oftentimes preceded by severe shaking chills? If yes, then it is bacterial. Has the fever waxed and waned over weeks, such as a chronic infection or as subacute infectious endocarditis or tuberculosis? Does the pulse rate go up in the standard ratio of ten beats to one degree increase of temperature? In typhoid fever, the pulse goes up slightly but not to the ratio of ten to one. Does the patient feel ill with the fever? Oftentimes drug reactions do not cause one to feel ill. Is the fever high, intermittently spiking, suggestive of a blocked duct? As stated earlier, gallbladder and renal blockages are causes of this type of fever; this is important in the elderly as oftentimes they may not show symptoms in these organ systems.

Did the patient start on a new medication? Recently started medicines are always suspect as causes of fever. Are there any joint or abdominal pains? That is, are there symptoms referable to a particular body system, such as joint, gastrointestinal, genitourinary, and so forth? Fevers can come from the gastrointestinal tract, and they may not be associated with infection (colitis, Crohn's disease). Similarly, joints may not be infected but the patient may have gout or a collagen disease (rheumatoid arthritis, scleroderma). Sometimes, diseases such as walking pneumonia may not have symptoms in the respiratory system.

If your symptoms were serious enough to bring you to your doctor or to the emergency room, then you should expect a laboratory evaluation. A white blood cell count can usually indicate whether there is an infection versus an allergic reaction or whether the infection is viral or bacterial. If a patient is suffering from a serious bacterial infection, the white blood cell count will usually be elevated (perhaps not in infants and the elderly). This will be accompanied by what physicians call a shift to the left (that is, immature forms of leukocytes will be found in the blood specimen, as the mature cells are being used up to fight the infection). Associated with this, test results will show a lowering of the amount of lymphocytes in the serum. A test will almost never find eosinophils (white blood cells are basically comprised of leukocytes, lymphocytes, and eosinophils) in the serum of patients with serious bacterial infections. These cells appear in allergic re-actions and certain tapeworm infestations. Their production is suppressed during an infection as the body produces cortisone as a response to an infec-tion. Cortisone suppresses the allergic response.

In some serious bacterial infections, but mostly in viral infections, the white blood cell count is suppressed. In infections such as ehrlichiosis, white blood cells as well as platelets are destroyed by the bacteria. So these infections are suspected routinely when patients present with febrile ill-nesses during the summer months and are found to have low white blood cell counts as well as low platelet counts.

In our modern age no one should be treated in an emergency room setting without obtaining a white blood cell count. More importantly, if a serious infection is suspected, no one should be treated without blood cultures being taken to identify the offending organism. One of my pa-tients went to the emergency room, suffering from a high fever and was sent home with antibiotic therapy. Although he felt better for two days, he had a relapse. After evaluating him in my office and obtaining his workup from the hospital emergency room, it became obvious that they had diagnosed a urinary tract infection as the cause of his fever. A high fever is usually not a sign of a simple urinary tract infection, and what they should have done was obtain a blood culture. My patient really had a blockage of a ureter with an asymptomatic stone. His urinary tract infec-tion had spilled over into his bloodstream (sepsis) but went undetected because blood cultures were not done. As in many of the examples I use throughout this book, initially one can feel better with taking antibiot-ics, but the amount given orally will never be a match for a blood-borne infection.

So the history and physical examination, along with a white blood cell count will usually help point the physician in the right direction. A com-plete blood profile should also be done. This will indicate liver or kidney involvement. Obviously, other blood tests should be done, and other mo-dalities (x-ray, MRI, and so forth) should be considered where appropri-ate. Do not leave the emergency room, or for that matter, your physicians' office, until you understand what is wrong with you and that what you are told makes complete sense. And of course, if you are given antibiotics (after cultures are obtained), make sure you ask if the drug is in the same family as any you may be allergic to.

Upper respiratory infections include the sinuses, ears, and of course sore throats. If your sinuses or throat is sore for more than ten days, it is more than likely an allergy issue. Contrary to many myths, no one can look into a person's throat and know whether there is a strep infection or not. A throat culture is needed. Furthermore, the average person does not usually get strep throat: it is found mainly in children, parents of young children (unusually), and teachers of young children.

My daughter's boyfriend was told that he had strep throat while he was sick in the hospital. He is a law student and has no contact with children. Now there seems to be a joke somewhere here, perhaps about lawyers, but I am not going there, because lawyers are essential to the concept of this book (and who knows, he may wind up to be my son-in-law some day). Yes, a culture was taken and it did show *Streptococci*, but these were the normal kind that grow in our throats and not the dreaded group A, beta-hemolytic *Streptococci*. One has to question everyone, even the doctor who reads the culture incorrectly.

When is a cough more than just a cough? When your body and your doctor tell you so! Okay, perhaps this is not so venerably jokey. But the cough, a simple reflex contraction of the thoracic cavity to expel something irritating the throat or lungs, is one of the most misunderstood and misdiagnosed (by the layman, anyway) symptoms.

Coughing is considered indicative of many illnesses and conditions: inherent lung diseases (chronic obstructive pulmonary disease [COPD], asthma, etc.) or postnasal drips or allergies. Like most viral infections, viral pneumonia is a gradually progressive disease. Patients have malaise, weakness, and gradually develop cold symptoms and a cough. These symptoms may or not be associated with fever and usually do not produce greenish phlegm. Bacterial pneumonias, on the other hand, start off abruptly. One is healthy one day and the next has sudden chills, fever, and a productive (greenish phlegm) cough. The cough comes out of the blue (or green, in this case).

Patients with influenza can develop influenza pneumonia. They are sick with the flu and progressively get worse and worse over the next five to seven days. No antibiotics are indicated because this is a viral infection. This is in contraindicated with patients who are suffering from the flu and are gradually improving, when suddenly, four to seven days later, they develop chills, a new fever, and a productive cough. This is bacterial super-infection on top of a viral infection (the flu), and it does require treatment with antibiotics and perhaps hospitalization.

Fevers that occur immediately after surgery (the first day or two) are usually due to atelectasis (inadequate aeration of the lungs, causing them to "stick" together), an inflammation at the intravenous site, or a urinary tract infection, especially if the patient has an indwelling catheter. Wound infections, pulmonary embolisms, and pneumonias do not kick in for a few more days.

Neurologic infections are very serious and may be accompanied by headache, inability to move one's neck, or pain while trying to bend one's neck. They may be a consequence of another infection (severe sinusitis). The old adage if you have pneumonia and septicemia, meningitis is soon to follow still holds true. Patients who have meningitis should be started on antibiotics within an hour of being seen in an emergency room.

FOOD POISONING SIGNS AND PREVENTION

Depending on the type of food poisoning, symptoms can begin anywhere from a few hours to several days after eating contaminated food. The typical symptoms include abdominal pain, diarrhea, vomiting, and fever. Some forms of food poisoning will have vomiting without fever. And one of the most dangerous types, botulism, attacks the nervous system and exhibits signs of paralysis.

Signs/Symptoms of Specific Food Poisoning

Different types of food poisoning present with specific signs or symptoms:

- *Staphylococcus* preformed toxins: symptoms start within the first four hours after a meal: be especially suspicious if the meal included ham, poultry, mayonnaise-based salads, creamy pastries, fried rice, or vegetables.
- *Clostridium perfringens*: illness occurs ten to fourteen hours after a meal: be especially suspicious if the meal consisted of Mexican food, gravy, beef, or poultry.
- *Salmonella*: symptoms typically include fever, abdominal cramps, diarrhea, headache, and sometimes vomiting, usually developing twelve to seventy-two hours after exposure to contaminated food. In those with

poor underlying health or weak immune systems, the bacteria can enter the bloodstream and cause infections, which can sometimes be life-threatening. These symptoms, along with loss of appetite, can last for several days. Dehydration, especially among infants, can be severe.

- *Escherichia coli*: symptoms often begin within three to four days, but can occur up to eight days after becoming infected. *E. coli* is the cause of most traveler's diarrhea. Some people have no symptoms. Nevertheless, they can still pass the infection to others. Common signs and symptoms include diarrhea, abdominal cramping, nausea, dehydration, low-grade or no fever, and in extreme cases, hemolytic uremic syndrome (HUS), a serious complication that can cause kidney failure, seizures, and even death. Because it can take eight days for symptoms to start, most patients get sick either on their return trip or when they get home.
- *Shigella*: symptoms of shigellosis typically begin a day or two after exposure to contaminated substances. One of the most common signs is diarrhea, often bloody. Other symptoms can include abdominal cramps and fever.
- *Trichinosis*: symptoms can be mild (including nausea, diarrhea, vomiting, fatigue, fever, abdominal discomfort, itchy skin, and headache), to more severe symptoms of extreme versions of the above, as well as chills, eye swelling, aching joints and muscles, difficulty coordinating movement, and heart and breathing problems. The degree of severity can relate to the quantity of parasites consumed in the meat. Mild cases are often believed to be due to the flu or another common illness and are not properly diagnosed. But be advised, trichinosis has been on the rise lately, especially in areas where there are large pig farms. In addition, bear meat has also been shown to be infested with trichinosis.[2]

General treatment of food poisoning, except botulism, deals mainly with preventing dehydration by putting back the fluids and electrolytes lost through vomiting and diarrhea. Dehydration is more common in young children, the elderly, and people taking diuretics. Drink plenty of electrolyte-replacing sports drinks. In severe cases, physicians will prescribe intravenous fluids.

There have been many references in this book to *Clostridium difficile*. This gas-forming organism is normally present in our intestine and is a normal part of our bowel flora. Under certain circumstances it grows to significant pathogenic importance, especially when patients are placed on broad-spectrum antibiotics. It can cause significant illness and even death. If you or someone you know is taking an antibiotic and develops diarrhea and abdominal cramping, be concerned about a super infection with clostridia. My friend was recently hospitalized and was being treated with one week of intravenous antibiotic therapy. Fortunately I happened to be visiting when he suddenly got severe cramping abdominal pain and ran off to the bathroom with explosive diarrhea. This is the classic presentation of illness due to *Clostridium difficile*. I immediately went to one of the physicians caring for him, who turned out to be a fellow infectious disease specialist. I told her my concerns and observations regarding a clostridial infection and asked if she would honor my request and do the test that would identify the presence of that particular organism. "Of course," she said. That was on a Sunday. Perhaps due to the continuation of his diarrhea and cramping, the test was finally ordered on Wednesday. Maybe the doctor forgot to order the test or perhaps she did not like being told how to do her job. The test was positive and finally my friend was then appropriately treated. Hopefully, your doctor will be more responsive. Once clostridial infection is diagnosed, another antibiotic must be prescribed for its treatment.

PRESCRIPTION

- If you have an infection, you must find out which kind. That requires a culture, whether it be your urine, blood, throat, stool, or whatever.
- No antibiotic therapy should ever be started without being preceded by a culture.
- Make sure the drug you are given is not in the same family as the one you may be allergic to, ask the doctor and the pharmacist.
- No injection or pill gets into you without your requesting why.
- Revisit the need for use of the drug after the culture returns.
- Determining the extent or depth of the infection will determine the route (oral or intravenous) and length of therapy.
- If you have more than the routine infection, ask for an infectious disease consultation.
- Your treatment should involve your PCP, especially if you have a surgical infection.

HOW TO MAINTAIN SOME SANITY
IN THE MENTAL HEALTH SYSTEM

PSYCHOLOGISTS, PSYCHIATRISTS, AND PSYCHOANALYSIS

Psychiatrists and most analysts have an M.D. (*Medicinea Doctor*; Latin for "teacher of medicine")[1] degree. Thus, only psychiatrists and M.D. analysts can prescribe medication. Recently, psychologists who go through more specific training have attempted to get the right to prescribe. It is possible that others who practice psychotherapy, such as counselors and social workers, may want to have that ability in the future. Without being biased, I feel that M.D.-trained therapists seem to have a more profound overall understanding of the human organism, mind and body, as well as their interconnections, than do other trained therapists. This is not meant to demean other therapists, as I refer patients equally to them as well. It is important to recognize that there are many conditions in the mental health field that receive better treatment either with medication alone or, as with many cases, a combination of medication and talk therapy. In the more severe cases of mental decompensation (i.e., psychosis, manic depressive disorder, and severe anxiety), medication is a very important part of the treatment. I will comment later on the place of electroconvulsive therapy (ECT) in the treatment program for severe conditions.

Not every area of emotional or behavioral conditions secondary to learn-ing difficulties or hyperactivity is treated in only one way. Understandably, different approaches claim success with different methods. However, some consensus does exist for certain disorders of behaviors seen in chil-dren and adolescents.

As a general rule, when one sees a non-M.D. therapist, he or she should inquire whether the therapist has any bias with regard to the use of medica-tion. One should also inquire if the therapist is able to refer to two or three medically trained people during treatment if it should become necessary.

PROBLEMS AND SOLUTIONS

In Choosing a Therapist

It is important to inquire regarding the bias of the therapist because some non-M.D. therapists have a negative bias toward medications, believing in many instances that all conditions, except schizophrenia, can be handled by talk therapy alone. On the other hand, there are some psychiatrists who rely only on medication with little attention to psychodynamics and, therefore, do not deal comfortably with talk therapy. I believe that one should choose to consult with a therapist who has no bias but possesses a balanced recognition of the value of multiple approaches.

In general, issues of diagnosis and medication are overlapping ones in both general medicine and psychiatry. A clear and correct diagnosis helps to get to the proper treatment quickly and successfully. If needed, the correct medication, in an adequate dosage can contribute to a good outcome. In the ensuing discussion, some repetition is inevitable. Viewing treatment issues according to demographic and age grouping is helpful and insightful.

In Treating Children

In this age category, most therapists are presented with behavior and learning disabilities. More commonly, these revolve around the diagnoses of attention deficit disorder (ADD) and attention deficit with hyperactivity disorder (ADHD). Both of these conditions are most often detected in the school setting, although many parents may observe these conditions with-out being aware of the problem in clear terms. They may attribute their child's behavior to a passing phase with a comment that he or she is "just a child." When ADD or ADHD is not dealt with early on, teachers will often find that these students have more behavioral issues, their learning is poorer, and they are more easily distracted than their classmates. For that matter, their behavior can also cause unwelcome distractions among the other children.

Nowadays, more teachers are aware of these manifestations than years ago, and they do not deal with these children as bad children. Often, it seems that when ADD or ADHD children are dealt with as bad children, they become more angry and withdrawn, and their more negative symptoms worsen, adding to their already lowered self-esteem.

The use of stimulants for these conditions has been a great help in moderating the above behaviors and subsequent sequelae. However, some controversy has developed between pro and con groups. Some are convinced that behavior modification can do the job of ameliorating these conditions. Some are fearful that early use of stimulants, such as methylphenidate (Ritalin), may later lead to other drug use. There is no evidence for this concern.[2] Being able to seat children within a classroom in such a way that they are not distracted, while also preventing them from distracting others, can be very helpful. But the success of the stimulants has been very clear.

There have been some suggestions that the use of stimulants in early childhood may lead to the stunting of growth, but in this very small group, growth accelerates back to normal when the drugs are stopped.[3] A small percentage of children appear to naturally outgrow these conditions, but we are not sure whether their self-esteem has been permanently affected. Interestingly, I had a 47-year-old physicist consult with me after he had read an article on ADHD and felt that he fell into that diagnosis. A trial of methylphenidate greatly improved his capacity to focus and remain in long conferences without having to get up and leave. The ADD part is clearly helped with stimulants. There is less spacing-out and more capacity to stick to academic learning. Many of these children can focus for long periods of time watching television or using building toys.

In Treating Adolescents

In adolescence, in addition to experimentation with drugs and/or alcohol, there can be a serious issue with depression. Depression can be triggered in this vulnerable age group by demands of the age and peer pressures, as well as stresses with parents at home, with teachers at school, heightened self-consciousness, sexual pressures, and early expressions of manic depression.

Psychotherapy and medication have been used for many years in this age group and have often been effective.[4] Suicide and suicidal ideation in a few cases have been linked to certain classes of antidepressants. Patients in this age group need to be closely monitored when they are started on this class of drugs. Early manic depressive behavior is a bit more difficult to diagnose in this stage. Some evidence of manic depression has been found in preteen years. Early diagnosis of this condition can help prevent the more severe expressions of this genetic disorder as well as the need for hospitalization for dangerous behavior, leading possibly to death.

In Treating Late Adolescents: 17 to 22 Years of Age

This age group sees the onset of, as well as a higher incidence of, schizophrenia with its many manifestations. Here again, those with this diagnosis will require medication that can soften the severe expression of this disorder and possibly mute some of the sequelae. A sudden onset of mania can be misdiagnosed as schizophrenia. Lithium has become the main drug for stabilizing mania and perhaps modifying the depression that often is seen oscillating with mania at various intervals.

Lithium has to be monitored carefully, as do other antimanic drugs. Toxicity can develop with lithium when higher drug levels develop in the blood. This can happen during a fever, when the associated dehydration can cause a rapid increased lithium concentration, leading to toxicity. Tremors and disorientation may ensue. Hydration and the discontinuance of lithium during this circumstance are essential. Thyroid imbalance can be a common side effect of lithium use, and thus it needs to be monitored. The combination of lithium and alcohol is also a problem in these teens and young adults.

Usually, schizophrenia is mainly handled as a medical psychiatric condition. All medicines, however, have side effects, including weight gain, tremors, Parkinson-like movements, disorientation, onset of prediabetes, or liver abnormalities. So, again, monitoring the patient during treatment is of utmost importance.

In Treating during the Middle Years

Rarely do we see the onset of schizophrenia or manic depression in middle age. At this point, depressive illness can become more prominent.

Often, it seems that mild to moderate depression is well handled by combining antidepressants and talk therapy. More severe depressions may need hospitalization if hints of suicide are detected. In some severe depression, formally labeled psychotic depression, and often with clear suicidal ideation, electroconvulsive therapy (ECT) can be effective. Popularly called shock therapy in the past, ECT is usually given in short courses of six to eight treatments. This is usually effective in bringing a patient out of this severe depression. If treated otherwise, this condition could take six months or more to resolve.

ECT has been wrongly accused of being barbarous and dangerous. Modern ECT techniques cause very low side effects or dangers. There is some loss of memory, which most often is regained in the ensuing months. The most dangerous period after recovery from severe depression, however, is when the patient appears superficially well. This is the time that suicide can often occur; therefore, careful monitoring of the patient is necessary for several months following treatment.

In Treating in the Geriatric Stage

In the geriatric age group, depression is the main problem. This condition can be treated as noted previously. But added difficulties arise here because of the multiple medications that are used in this more sickness-prone population. Many elderly suffer from heart disease, chronic obstructive pulmonary disease, arthritis, urinary problems, and so forth. Those that suffer with these conditions often take medications that can conflict with psychotropic medications. Antidepressants may affect urination and can cause constipation as well as some disorientation (in an already borderline mentated state). Paranoid ideation may be stimulated by some medications. Again, it is possible that this use of other medications to counteract the paranoid ideation may have unwanted side effects. Remember, researching all of the known side effects of medication and keeping an eye out for them is not only the responsibility of the treating physician but the family as well.

The Role of the Family

Family and close friends are most important. As noted above, medications need careful monitoring and those closest to the patient are in the best position to note any of these, at times subtle, changes. With children, adolescents, and the geriatric populations, monitoring is essential, and, therefore, if a patient does not bring family or friends to the sessions, it can be a serious detriment to treatment as well as their well-being.

ADDED CAVEATS

Psychiatry presents many of the same problems of general medicine particularly in the area of medications.

Adolescents are classically resistant to following orders, and, often, their reports on their intake of medication and following of prescription dosage are faulty. Thus, this age group also needs special monitoring.

Care must be taken not to rapidly decrease the dosage of tranquilizers because this may lead to withdrawal phenomenon—rebound hyperanxiety and headaches. Conversely, rapid reduction of antidepressants can lead to anxiety and, at times, disorientation.

That being said, many of the causes of malpractice in psychiatry are similar to those in general medicine. Misdiagnosis and therefore ensuing mistreatment have been covered by the Institute of Medicine's Chasm Series and reported by Benjamen Grasso in his article, which reveals that drug errors and misdiagnosis errors are similar in rates with general medicine.[5]

To further complicate issues, almost all psychiatric medicines have severe side effects. Every one of my severely mentally ill patients (and many who are not that ill) is either suffering from abnormal muscular twitching, slurred speech, or abnormal walking. If you were to read the *Physicians Desk Reference*, many of these psychotropic drugs can cause increases in depression or initiate suicide ideation. It seems to me that we do not yet have a handle on prescribing these drugs. However, it is a far cry better than years ago.

Many of these drugs require constant monitoring (of drug levels) because they are prescribed at near toxic dosages. There are also metabolic side effects that can occur, such as liver disease, blood dyscrasias, and cardiac arrhythmias. All of these side effects require frequent blood analysis (and at times electrocardiogram evaluations). If your doctor is not monitoring you, at least on a quarterly basis, you may want to seek other help.

Furthermore, each drug class has specific side effects that should be Googled and family members should monitor these side effects.

As a general rule, all therapists should be chosen for their knowledge, experience, and empathy. These attributes lead to the most likelihood of success. This is easily said in our atmosphere of a medical crisis, where some insurance policies do not cover mental illness or may not cover many psychiatrists. To add to this mix, many psychiatrists do not take insurance because the payments may be too little or there is too much paperwork involved per patient.

Psychiatrists can also make mistakes, both in diagnosis, medication, and dosage. As with hospitals and PCP offices, many mistakes arise from indecipherable handwriting, all calling for triple checking on everyone's part.

PRESCRIPTION

- It may be dangerous to immediately cease taking psychiatric drugs because of potential significant withdrawal side effects. You will need the advice and assistance of a competent physician.
- It is very important that these medications not be left around as they have been shown to be lethal if ingested by toddlers.
- Psychiatrists, like all physicians, have to be questioned as to why they are proposing a particular treatment.
- It is important to keep notes, to keep your own records, or to keep an independent diary of what happens at each visit with your psychiatrist.
- It makes sense to keep records of what medications you have been taking, along with changes in dosage and changes in drugs. All too often patients present with new unusual symptoms and upon careful review of the side effects of their psychotropic medications (and there are so many), one can easily find the reason. Usually, any addition of a medication preceding the new symptoms is the presumed cause until proven otherwise.

III

THE HOSPITAL AND MAJOR PROCEDURES

(12)

HOSPITAL OUTPATIENT VISITS AND HOW TO MAKE SURE YOU ACTUALLY GET OUT!

I learned a long time ago that minor surgery is when they do the operation on someone else, not you.

—Bill Walton[1]

Thirty-five years ago, a local Westchester hospital had three or four general surgeons. They were all quite busy but always had room to see another patient. These three or four surgeons were able to adequately service all of the patients in the hospital's catchment area (the surrounding area that supplied the patients). Ten years later, something very strange occurred. Twelve to fifteen new surgeons decided to enter into practice there. Guess what happened? It seemed that while drawing from the same population, which did not change dramatically, all eighteen or so surgeons became very busy. How was that possible?

Is it possible that where there was a surgeon available, reasons for surgery were found? How else could one explain the dramatic increase in surgical procedures? To a hammer, everything looks like a nail. This sudden demand for operating room time by so many surgeons stressed the small operating theater to the max. More operating suites were added, but that still was not enough. Instead of the prior calm and relatively short waiting period for surgical procedures, now patients had lengthy waits until their surgery could be scheduled. The patients who had to wait the longest were those who needed surgery that took many hours. Why tie up a room for hours when you can do two or three procedures during the same time period? Emergencies were, of course, always accommodated. To add to this increased demand, approximately twelve new gastroenterologists were added to the staff. Similar to the surgical explosion, gastroenterologists were using precious outpatient space for endoscopies, colonoscopies, and other procedures that were now mandated to be done in a hospital setting.

Then the insurance companies added their two cents. I noticed that many insurance companies seemed to have decided that many surgical procedures could be done without hospitalization, and they often refused to pay hospitals for overnight stays. If you had your gallbladder removed, you were homeward bound that very same night. The term "drive-through mastectomy" entered our lexicon because women were being sent home immediately after their mastectomies. These insurance companies and HMOs were now dictating how, and how long, physicians, in this case surgeons, should treat their patients. Then along came the outpatient medical surgical unit. These were free-standing buildings loaded with operating room suites, colonoscopy rooms, stress testing equipment, and so forth. The problem with this, however, was that there seemed to be no change in the complication rate of surgery or any of the other same-day procedures.

For example, if 10 percent of patients were to develop a postsurgical infection, they would develop the infection at home, after being discharged from hospital care where they would have been under twenty-four-hour observation of trained medical personnel. If patients were going to develop intestinal obstruction after surgery, or if something was accidentally cut and didn't show up for twelve to twenty-four hours, the patient would be home before that occurred, now without medical supervision. The sooner one finds a complication, the better chance there is to fix the problem. Under these circumstances, the odds of such a timely discovery were obviously decreased. Elective gallbladder surgery is presently done in one day, and the patient is usually kept overnight. Some outpatient surgical units let their gallbladder patients out the same day. I reviewed a case recently of one such patient who was sent home *four hours* after having his gallbladder removed laparoscopically. He awoke in the middle of the night with moderately intense abdominal pain and was jaundiced by the time he was brought to the emergency room that morning. His common bile duct had been accidentally severed during the preceding day's surgery and it didn't make itself known until hours after he was home.

The thing to understand is that, all things being equal, the same errors occur whether you are at an outpatient facility or being treated at the hospital. One must, therefore, be much more alert to nuances and symptoms that may arise after surgery. Lori recently had outpatient surgery for removal of a cyst on her elbow. She was repeatedly asked about her allergies prior to surgery. She informed at least four personnel of her allergies to iodine. Approximately two and a half hours after surgery, she developed severe itching under the cast that kept her elbow from bending. The burning and itching became so severe that she had to return to the outpatient clinic. It turned out that Betadine (an iodine preparation) was used preoperatively to sterilize her skin. The cast was removed, her skin was cleansed, and a new cast was applied. In this case, the result was not life-threatening. But it certainly could have been. Some allergic reactions can kill you.

There certainly is a convenience to going home and recuperating after surgery. Many people decide to do so, even if there is a minor complication during surgery. After all, the dangers of staying in the hospital might be far worse than taking our chances at home! We could be given the wrong medicine, the wrong test, or catch one of those insidious hospital-acquired infections. But with this added convenience comes an increased responsibility to both the medical practitioner and you, the proactive patient. Since you cannot necessarily control how the medical team will perform, you must take things into your own hands. You must be more observant, both by making sure you are not being given any medications you are allergic to and by immediately reporting any new symptoms or changes that may arise before, during, and after the procedure.

If possible, I recommend having your outpatient procedure first thing in the morning. The staff tends to be more alert, less tired, and not watching the clock. The operating suite is also truly sterile before the first surgical case of the day. In addition, the odds of being able to stay and be observed all day, rather than being asked to leave a few hours later, are greatly increased. Most state laws require that you be accompanied by an adult that day, as well as be driven home by someone other than yourself. Your chaperone should write down everything the doctor and nurse suggests because you are likely to still be groggy afterward and unlikely to accurately remember what they told you. They should get all emergency phone numbers and know specifically whom to call if there is a complication or a question.

Most of us are told to see the doctor in ten to fourteen days for suture removal or follow-up visits. If you are getting a procedure, such as endoscopy or colonoscopy, you will likely have biopsies taken and sent to the lab for a pathologist to examine. In that case, you will want to follow-up for results. Don't assume that the doctor's office will call you, even if your results are positive. Many patients have discovered problems too late because of that erroneous assumption! Regardless of results, having a follow-up visit will allow you to discuss the findings in-depth and ask any residual questions. I would demand my first follow-up within one to two days, when complications usually show themselves. I can't tell you how many times patients have tried to describe an abdominal cramp or "gas" pain over the telephone when a look is really worth more than a thousand words. Those supposed gas pains may be nothing and are often brushed off by the office staff, nurse, and sometimes even the physician. How often have I called a specialist or surgeon to discuss a mutual patient that I was seeing who was having a complication? "Well, the doctor is in surgery," responds the nurse, "perhaps I can help?" Nurses are great and are needed, but during crunch time, I would rather have their boss on the phone. All too often I have seen their pooh-poohing of seemingly innocuous symptoms as having caused serious delays in proper treatment. As a patient, I would take the nurse's opinion but still insist that I get a call back from the physician. I would rather be examined early on and then be told directly by the surgeon that there is nothing to worry about. In fact, I suggest that you make a deal with the surgeon prior to surgery. Make sure that the surgeon will speak with you daily for two to four days after the procedure. If you make this arrangement upfront, you are more likely to get a timely response than if you wait and just wing it. Of course, make sure you are seen immediately if you feel uncomfortable or if something just doesn't feel right. You are paying for the surgery and deserve your surgeon's attention. If you are not seen, then quickly get a second opinion.

Remember, while an outpatient procedure is generally less complicated than inpatient surgeries, many complications can still arise. Don't assume that just because the surgical staff gets you in and out that you can treat the procedure as if it is no big deal while you go on with your life as if nothing happened. Take the time to prepare your handy list of questions as well as any medications and allergies to medications you may have. Make sure you get all your questions answered sufficiently before your procedure. Then stay alert to every medication they are giving you and every procedure they are performing. As I suggested, I recommend that you schedule these operations first thing in the morning to get the staff and facilities at their freshest. And then, if possible, stay there for the day to be observed. The extra time and energy that you put in will be one of the best investments that you have ever made, yielding better care and more peace of mind.

One of the most common outpatient experiences for those of us over 50 years old is a colonoscopy. Believe it or not, I have seen many people saved just by having this simple, painless, procedure, when it was done routinely. Therefore, because of its importance, let me run you through this common procedure. The day before, you will be told to go on a liquid diet and then later that evening you will take some form of an intestinal cleanser. Staying up all night with cramps and diarrhea is actually the worst part of the colonoscopy. Remember, your goal is to be the first patient being done that morning, when you will be assured that the colonoscope will be sterile. On the morning of the procedure, you are probably tired and grumpy from staying up all night and you will be asked to strip down and change into a hospital gown that allows access to your rectum.

Try to have the procedure done in the hospital or at the medical surgical outpatient unit and not at the doctor's office. If there is a complication or perforation, you want to be where the surgeons are and not have to await an ambulance trip. The anesthesiologist will start an intravenous line. Make sure they open up the line to allow fluid to drip into you. At this point, you and your chaperone have already informed the doctors of your allergies, problems with anesthesia, and the medications you have taken. If you have a significant heart murmur, artificial joint, or other hardware in your body, you will need a prophylactic antibiotic, which will be given to you via your intravenous line by the anesthesiologist. Similarly, be aware that if you are on warfarin (Coumadin) or cortisone, your doses would have been adjusted days before this procedure. Once the drip starts, the intravenous anesthesia will kick in and you will be in the "twilight zone." You will probably not remember anything from this point on, including whatever the gastroenterologist tells you on your way out the door to go home. Hopefully, you will be allowed to stay two to three hours after the procedure, just to make sure there wasn't a perforation. A perforation is not a good thing, and it may take a few hours to make itself apparent.

Your chaperone may be told that the test was perfectly normal. Sometimes, because there might have been two or three areas of inflammation, your chaperone might also be informed that biopsies had to be taken, but 99.9 percent of the time these are normal, so sometimes it seems like they are ordered just to increase the price of the procedure. In a similar manner, it seems that sometimes cardiologists who perform angiographies earn an enormous amount of extra money for putting in a stent in your coronary artery, even if it is not needed. This extra procedure puts more money in the cardiologist's pocket above and beyond the money earned for the angiography.

Are more stents and colonic biopsies done than should be? I feel that there are. Do these extra procedures increase the chances of complications? I feel that they do. Should you know the integrity and level of competence of your procedure giver? I have observed that the busier the practitioner is, the closer the correlation to a decrease in the "extra" work. I am not saying that biopsies, stents, and whatever other procedures there are, are not needed. Indeed, many times they save lives. But I am saying that there can be a certain amount of excess. Just be aware, ask questions, and get second opinions.

Lastly, your chaperone must be very clear on whom to call if there is a questionable problem once you leave. Will your doctor be available? If not, who is the covering physician? Until when and where will you be able to find them? Perhaps it is not a good idea to have your procedure on Friday if the doctor will be away for the weekend.

PRESCRIPTION

- Before you commit to any surgical procedure, do your due diligence to make sure you actually need it: ask your doctor exactly why you need it, what your alternative options are, and what will happen if you don't do it.
- Get a second opinion if you are still uncertain.
- Research the surgeon's and/or hospital's track record with that particular procedure and research the procedure online.
- Make a list of all your questions and concerns and get the answers you need from your doctor before you commit to the surgery and on the day of the procedure.

- Schedule the outpatient procedure early in the morning.
- Pay close attention to any medications you are given, making sure you are not allergic to any of them.
- If you are feeling anxious about the procedure, tell your surgeon, doctor, and the medical staff that you have read about all the medical errors that can occur and you are feeling uneasy. Just like in the emergency room, that can keep them all on their toes.
- Ask to stay for the day, or at least several hours, under observation.
- Stay aware of any new symptoms that arise once you are home.
- If you have a friend or family member that can attend to you, let them know all the pertinent information about your operation, and ask them to keep an eye out for any unusual changes in your condition.

13

HOSPITAL STAYS:
AS DANGEROUS AS A WAR ZONE?

A hospital is no place to be sick.

—Samuel Goldwyn[1]

An elderly woman called a particular hospital and said, "Hello, darling, I'd like to talk with the person who gives the information regarding your patients. I want to know if the patient is getting better, doing as expected, or getting worse."

"What is the patient's name and room number?" the nurse at the station asked over the phone.

"Sarah Finkel, in room 719," the woman responded.

"Oh, yes. Mrs. Finkel is doing very well," the nurse said. "In fact, she's had two full meals, her blood pressure is fine, and her blood work just came back as normal. She's going to be taken off the heart monitor in a couple of hours and if she continues this improvement, Dr. Cohen is going to send her home Tuesday at twelve o'clock."

"Thank God!" the woman said. "That's fantastic, darling! That's wonderful news!'

"From your enthusiasm, I take it you must be a close family member or a very close friend," the nurse said.

"I'm Sarah Finkel in 719!" the woman snapped. "My doctor doesn't tell me *bupkes*!"

Hospitals come in many sizes: big, small, private, community, tertiary (specializing in heart surgery, transplantation, etc.), university, and teaching. University and teaching hospitals will give lots of attention to patients, but that attention may consist of repetitive examinations by students, interns, and residents. You can be sure you will have an abundance of specialists available, and they will be preceded by a lot of residents and fellows in training. Conversely, the more rural the hospital, the smaller the hospitals tend to be. Often there are fewer specialists on attending staffs in these smaller, more rural, hospitals, as they are catering to a smaller community of patients. Obviously you want the hospital you pick to be near your home, which may limit your choice. But whatever hospital you choose, big or small, urban or rural, the most important thing to keep in mind is that this is the primary breeding ground of the third leading cause of death in the United States—and the core subject of this book—medical malpractice. To beat a dead horse (one that probably died of natural causes, since animals hopefully suffer less malpractice than humans), medical error is a true public health hazard, a pandemic in a very real sense. It is a danger on the same level as smoking, auto accidents, and pollution. In fact, it occurs in 20 percent of all hospitalized patients.[2] That is one in every five patients! So, in the final analysis, choosing the best, and safest, hospital may take priority over choosing the closest.

We covered some of the causes of medical malpractice, which can vary based on many factors. However, they can be categorized as follows:

- Lack of skill of a doctor.
- Overworked and exhausted medical practitioners.
- Injury caused by employees of the doctor or hospital.
- Use of unsafe, untested, or inappropriate drugs or medicines.
- Unsafe hospital procedures or equipment. This includes defective and toxic products, and failure to recall defective defibrillators and pacemakers.
- Hospital-acquired infection. This is one of the worst culprits, yet it is not normally viewed as malpractice. However, considering that the hospital's main function is to make you better, having conditions that lead to such widespread infection should be considered medical error. As a comparison, if you brought your car in to be repaired and it was running worse as a result of being in the shop, that would be considered the error of the mechanics, right?

The first report sounding the alarm on malpractice was published in 1999 by the Institute of Medicine ([IOM], part of the National Academy of Sciences). At that time it was reported, as already mentioned in the Introduction, that 100,000 patients die annually in American hospitals, and these deaths were attributable to preventable medical errors. The cost to individuals, their families, and society at large for these errors was estimated at $20 to $30 billion annually. In some cases, these figures have been surpassed. One study in Kentucky showed that 1,000 patients die annually in their hospitals due to preventable medical malpractice events.[3] The cost borne in Kentucky by residents, patients and their families, and the community at large was greater than $300 million annually. A report on New York hospitals revealed an average of twenty-seven instances, per hospital, of invasive procedures performed on the wrong patient in a one-year period.[4] The same review of Florida hospitals found an average of eight patients per hospital.[5]

Hospitals account for a significant amount of medical malpractice because of the invasive procedures performed. A little-known 1974 study of California hospitals showed that 0.8 percent of hospitalized patients were injured by negligence in the hospital, and, ironically, the patients were in the hospital *because of negligent care by their doctors.*[6] Did you follow that? Patients had to go to the hospital because their doctors had injured them! That amounted to 250,000 injured patients. Another study of New York State hospitalized patients in 1984 revealed 1 percent of patients that year were injured by negligence. This caused the demise of a quarter of these patients. That is a total of 234,000 injuries and 56,000 killed.[7] Yes, I said "killed." Not intentionally, of course. But I think it is important not to soften the blow of these statistics by saying "they died due to complications." No, they were killed by medical error.

Has a different ring to it, doesn't it? Hopefully it is more of a wail than a ring, like an alarm going off. Interestingly, only one malpractice claim was (and is still) made for every 7.6 hospital-induced negligent injuries.

HealthGrades, Inc., originally found that 195,000 patients in the United States died due to potentially preventable "in-hospital" medical errors every year (for 2000, 2001, and 2002).[8] That is even worse than the opening statistics of this book. That is *more* than one jumbo jet full of people crashing and killing everyone on board—every day of the year. In fact, it is the equivalent of 390 jumbo jets full of people dying each year due to preventable "in-hospital" medical errors. The HealthGrades report was published in July 2004.

It cited the 1999 Institute of Medicine's report as too low (90,000 deaths was too low; that is us Americans, always trying to top ourselves). Health-Grades is the leading health care ratings organization, providing ratings and profiles of hospitals, nursing homes, and physicians. Millions of consumers and many of the nation's largest employers, health plans, and hospitals rely on HealthGrades's independent ratings.[9]

The IOM's 1999 report called for a 50 percent reduction in errors over the next five years. Unfortunately, this error rate has increased instead of decreased. Some of the IOM's recommendations were:

- Keeping patients safe (this one was a real revelation!).
- Transforming the work environment of nurses.
- Identifying solutions to problems in hospitals, nursing homes, and other health care organizations' work environments that threaten patient safety through their effect on nursing care. (Why didn't I think of that?)
- Achieving a new standard of care.
- Giving a detailed plan to facilitate data standards.
- Establishing a national standard.
- Creating comprehensive patient safety programs in health care organizations.

One major cause of medical malpractice causing morbidity and mortality in hospital patients, as previously indicated, is infection. Approximately 3 million hospitalized patients a year, 10 percent, will contract hospital-related infections. According to the Centers for Disease Control and Prevention, 90,000 of these patients who contract in-hospital infections will die every year.[10] Not all of these are caused by medical malpractice, but the majority of them seem to be. The recent increase in antibody-resistant bacteria and the mounting cost of caring for these patients add $4.5 billion annually to our health care bill.

To further complicate matters, many physicians give antibiotics to potentially ill patients without first adequately culturing the infected area. Oftentimes surface bacteria are cultured rather than getting deep into a wound for a culture. This misuse of antibiotics can obscure an infection and fool the physician into thinking he or she used the right antibiotic, only to hide the more serious infection (such as that of the heart or bone). I have frequently had to tell patients to stop their course of antibiotics for a week or more in order to allow the proper culturing and identification of their infections.

The *Chicago Tribune* reported in 2002 that 75,000 Americans die yearly from hospital-acquired nosocomial (Greek for "our house") infections that were preventable.[11] They reported that not enough hand washing and changing of scrubs were the major causes. Interestingly, but, based on the logic of the medical industry so far, not surprisingly, since 1995, *American hospitals have pared down their cleaning staffs by close to 30 percent.*[12] Is it just me, or are things going in the opposite direction? It is like realizing you are driving on the wrong side of the freeway—so you speed up! Have we fallen down the rabbit hole and not realized it? A recent study showed that doctors washed their hands, in between seeing each patient, only 44 percent of the time if nobody was looking. If they knew they were being watched, then 61 percent washed up.[13]

Adding to the list of causes for medical malpractice is the growing shortage of nurses. Low nurse staffing directly affects patient outcomes, resulting in problems such as resistant urinary tract infections, shock, and gastrointestinal bleeding. This was reported in 2001 by a study done by Harvard and Vanderbilt professors. Studies show that patients in hospitals where nurses had heavier workloads also had a higher risk of dying. Each additional patient per nurse corresponds to a 7 percent increase in patient morbidity and deaths following complications. Nevertheless, nursing shortages persist.[14]

As this book was going to press HealthGrades issued two important studies reviewing 41 million Medicare patient records at 5,000 hospitals over a three-year period. The first study was the HealthGrades eleventh annual Hospital Quality Study. Based on the study, HealthGrades made available on their Web site quality ratings for all nonfederal hospitals in the country. Full reports on death rate trends in each of the fifty states are available in the study. And the report includes hospital death rates for the nation's fifteen largest metropolitan statistical areas.

The astounding revelation was that patients had a 70 percent lower chance of dying at the nation's top-rated hospitals compared with the lowest-rated hospitals. This was determined by studying seventeen procedures and conditions. While overall death rates declined slightly from 2005 to 2007, the nation's best-performing hospitals were able to reduce their death rates at a much faster rate than poorly performing hospitals, resulting in large state, regional, and hospital-to-hospital variations in the quality of patient care.

The study concluded that if all hospitals performed at the level of those five-star–rated hospitals, 237,420 Medicare deaths could have been prevented over that three-year period. That is to say 80,000 Medicare patients could have been saved every year. Large gaps persist between the best and the worst hospitals across all procedures and diagnoses studied. Five-star–rated hospitals had significantly lower risk-adjusted mortality across all three years studied. Across all procedures and diagnoses studied, there was a 70 percent lower chance of dying in a five-star–rated hospital compared to a one-star hospital (as noted above). However, across all procedures and diagnoses studied, there was a 50 percent lower chance of dying in a five-star hospital compared to the U.S. hospital average. Interestingly, the region with the lowest overall risk adjusted mortality rates was the east northcentral region (Illinois, Indiana, Michigan, Ohio, and Wisconsin). This region had the highest percentage of best performing hospitals, at 26 percent. Less than 7 percent of hospitals within the New England region were top performing hospitals. Out of the 5,000 hospitals studied by HealthGrades, how many hospitals do you think were considered five star? Twenty-five percent? Perhaps 20 percent? A mere 250 hospitals got the top rating. That is 5 percent of the hospitals. That does not include veteran's or military hospitals. No other federal hospitals were included, so the percentage of best care hospitals goes down to much less than 5 percent.[15]

The second study issued by HealthGrades was the fourth annual Patient Safety in American Hospitals Study. This study, like the previous one, used the same database of 41 million Medicare patients in 5,000 hospitals but during a different three-year period, from 2003 to 2005. The definition of patient safety for the study was "freedom from accidental injury due to medical care, or medical errors." They defined medical error as the failure of a planned action to be completed as intended or the use of a wrong plan to achieve an aim, including problems in practice, products, procedures, and systems.

The study showed that 1.16 million total patient safety incidents occurred in over 40 million hospitalizations in the Medicare population, which is almost a 3 percent incident rate. These incidents were associated with $8.6 billion of excess cost during 2003 through 2005. The total patient safety incident rate worsened by an additional 2 percent of incidents per 1,000 hospitalizations in 2005 compared to 2003. Of the 284,798 deaths that occurred among patients who developed one or more patient safety incidents, 247,662 were potentially preventable. Furthermore, Medicare beneficiaries that developed one or more patient safety incidents had a one in four chance of dying during the hospitalization during 2003 to 2005. As with the first study, there were wide, highly significant gaps in individual safety incidents and overall performance between the rated "Distinguished Hospitals for Patient Safety" and the bottom ranked hospital. Medicare patients in these Distinguished Hospitals for Patient Safety had a 40 percent lower occurrence of experiencing one or more safety incidents compared to the bottom ranked hospitals. Failure to rescue is shorthand for failure to prevent deterioration, such as death or permanent disability from an underlying illness. The patient safety indicators with the highest incidence rates were decubitus ulcers (bed sores), failure to rescue, and postoperative respiratory failure. If all hospitals performed at the level of the Distinguished Hospitals for Patient Safety, 206,298 patient safety incidents and 34,393 Medicare deaths could have been prevented while saving the United States $1.74 billion during the 2003 to 2005 study period.[16]

These reports did not cover other causes of injury to patients. One of the most common causes of injury, in a hospital setting, is falling. Patients fall because they are weak, feel faint, or become dizzy due to medications. Patients likely to fall are supposed to be identified at the time of admission and also reevaluated during their confinement. Are the patients stuporous, prone to falling, or dizzy? Do they have a history of falling? The hospital has to have a written manual that details a plan to prevent such falls. Should patients who are dizzy be restrained? At the very least, and what is recommended, is that patients who are prone to fall be placed in rooms just in front of the nurse's station, so that there can be better observation. At least 50 percent of physical injuries in hospitals occur from falling from either a bed or a chair. I once testified against a physician who ordered 20 milligrams of a sleep medication for his patient. The medication was ordered for an 80-year-old man who had difficulty in sleeping. The *Physicians' Desk Reference*, a guide for prescribing nurses and physicians, specifically states, in emboldened letters, that no more than 5 milligrams of that particular drug should be dispensed to any person over the age of 65. One would reason that if 5 milligrams would help put one to sleep, that 20 milligrams would do a better job? As it turns out, 10 or 20 milligrams does not do any better than 5 milligrams, it just increases the chances of unwanted side effects. In the case of this hallucinogenic drug, the incidence of dizziness and falling rises tremendously. Why this particular pharmaceutical company offers the higher dosages, knowing these facts (they print them in the *Physician's Desk Reference*), is beyond me. Why this particular physician ordered the 20 milligram dose (which is never indicated) is also beyond me. The elderly patient was found confused, lying on the hospital floor, with a fractured hip. His roommate stated that the patient was mumbling, fighting to get out of bed, tripped and fell. All this time, the roommate was ringing on his bedside call button, but nobody came to his aid.

The HealthGrades reports also did not cover medication errors, transfusion errors, or surgical errors, which I cover in another section of this book.

So that, my friends, is a snapshot of our current hospital situation in America. Not a pretty picture. Not a place that you would want to get a room at any time soon. Unfortunately, many people won't have that option. So what are you to do if you find yourself booking a stay at Sickness Central? First of all, don't go in scared. Despite all the negative statistics in this book, the fact still remains that plenty of people check in to hospitals and check out "all better." The minority of doctors and medical practitioners are responsible for the vast majority of malpractice incidents that occur. Nevertheless, to deny this growing problem would be like turning a blind eye to those jumbo jets crashing every day of the year. Remember, my intention is not to make you more frightened of the medical world, just more informed about it. The purpose of telling it like it is is to make sure that you do not take anything for granted and make sure that you take control of your health care experience.

Just as with the doctor visits, when you stay at the hospital, you are dealing with human beings: nurses, doctors, and other staff members who are dealing with their own issues—not the least of which are an abundance of bureaucratic, political, and workplace problems. I know that you are there because you are sick and need help. I know that they should be thinking only about how they can make your experience the best it can possibly be. I know that they should make sure that you heal in the quickest, most painless way possible. And I believe that, for most health care practitioners, that is what they wish, too. But, alas, that isn't the way things often are. And all of us physicians do make mistakes. So that once again puts the ball squarely in your court.

So what are you going to serve back to the medical practitioners working with you? As best as possible, you want to treat them with as much kindness and respect as you can. Thank them when they help you. Share personal things about yourself and seek to get to know them as well. The more personal you become with them, the closer your working health care relationship with them can be. The more you respect, validate, and appreciate them, the more they are likely to return the favor. Now is not the time to be proud. Swallow your pride. You can cough it up later, when you have made it out of the hospital, alive and well!

As always, do your research. If you have followed the guidance of this book, you investigated the hospital before you checked in, and you know the statistics for the particular procedure you are going in for. You have Googled until your fingers are sore. You have written out your questions and concerns, discussed them all with your doctor, and had every question answered completely. You have gotten a second—and sometimes even a third—opinion. You have brought along a friend or family member to crucial doctor appointments, before committing to the hospital stay, to be your objective witness.

Of course, depending on your location and insurance status, you may not have unlimited choice as to which hospital, doctor, or level of facilities you will have access to. This is, unfortunately, just the reality for some of us. Nevertheless, having a thorough knowledge of the hospital statistics, the doctor's track record, and a comprehensive list of questions and concerns that have been fully addressed—as well as an alert, proactive stance while in the hospital—will dramatically increase your chances of having a successful medical experience, regardless of the particular hospital and medical team you find yourself working with.

As you go through the experience of your stay, leading up to the particular procedure for which you are entering the hospital, make sure once again that every medication you take is the right one. Check and double check against any allergies you may have had. Ask the doctor exactly why you are taking it and what, if any, alternatives there are. What possible side effects and drug interactions are there? This goes for all tests as well. If the thought of being this assertive makes you want to curl up into a ball—snap out of it! But if you can't, enlist a good friend or caring family member to be your patient advocate. While you are staying in the hospital, as well as before, during, and after the day of any major procedures, it is also a good idea to have someone there to be an extra pair of eyes and ears.

Recently I received a phone call from a former classmate and similar specialist in infectious diseases. He had decided to practice medicine in Israel and is quite well known in his field. He had a problem. His only sibling, his sister, was in and out of a small community hospital in Long Island. He could not get the physician caring for his sister to speak with him and, to his dismay, she had already been in the hospital for a total of six weeks. The family had not even been told of any diagnosis. What he did know was that after she was in the hospital for about two weeks, she was sent home, where she would then collapse and have to be taken back to the hospital the next day. This cycle occurred on three separate occasions. Obviously, something was amiss. I spoke with the brother-in-law and obtained the physician's name and number. When I phoned, the doctor's nurse said that he does not speak to other doctors and would not come to the phone. That was a tip-off that he probably did not know what was wrong with my friend's sister. I next phoned the administrator of the hospital, who was in a meeting, and got the sympathy of his secretary. So far I am following the script I would have prescribed for you. One half hour later, the physician called. He was not apologizing, but he also had no clue as to what was going on. He shared no information with me so I called the husband and strongly suggested that, if it was okay with him, I would arrange for a transfer to a university hospital a half mile away. He was delighted. The chief of medicine at the university hospital agreed to the transfer, but there was a delay for a few days, as the insurance company objected to both the transfer and having to pay for the ambulance ride. On the day of transfer, the husband called to say that his wife had suffered a heart attack (so he was told) and needed heart surgery. What had actually happened was that she had had low-grade fevers, never had blood cultures taken, and was, unknowingly, suffering from endocarditis (an infection of the valves of the heart). She needed her heart valve repaired. If a doctor isn't forthcoming, or if he cannot come up with a reasonable answer, it is your duty to obtain a second opinion, sooner rather than later.

Of course if you are entering a hospital as the result of an accident, you may not have been able to do all the necessary preparation (the hopeful exception being if your accident occurs locally, and you have already scouted the hospitals in your area). If this is the case, fear not. As soon as you have presence of mind, that is the time to begin asking questions and making sure that you get answers. From that point on, question everything, kindly, but firmly. And get that patient advocate in there by your side.

PRESCRIPTION

- Research the hospitals in your area or wherever you may be staying for an extended period of time. Check statistics, doctors, specialists, and technical equipment quality.

- After reading the HealthGrades reports, it makes sense to be admitted to a five-star–rated hospital (which is usually also a Distinguished Hospital for Patient Safety) if it is possible. Odds are in your favor for a safer outcome and the chance you will leave that hospital in good shape. That doesn't mean that nothing can happen to you. One of my patients was recently in a five-star hospital. While in the intensive care unit the doctor told the nurse that my patient needed potassium. Instead of putting the potassium in the I.V. solution, she injected it directly into his vein. He screamed out because of severe burning and his blood pressure dropped to 50 as he went into shock. He did, however, survive.
- Get all your questions answered from your doctor, surgeon, anesthesiologist, and anyone else who will be on the medical team *before* entering the hospital and before any major procedures.
- To limit your susceptibility to acquiring hospital infections, make sure anyone who touches you washes their hands first. Infectious agents are commonly carried from one patient to another. In the old days before antibiotics, many unfortunate women died of puerperal sepsis (birthing mothers dying of rampant infection). Fortunately, a quite brilliant physician realized that midwives and physicians who were not washing their hands were probably passing the strep infection that was killing these women from one patient to the next. So he posted nurses, stationing them at the end of each ward. Their job was to blow a whistle at anyone who attempted entering a room without first washing his or her hands. This simple procedure ended the outbreak of a terrible human-induced disease and went on to save thousands of future lives.
- Cross-infection can occur frequently, such as when a nurse changes one catheter that is infected and then changes another without washing his or her hands. Be alert to these incidents and do not hesitate to point it out.
- Intravenous sites and catheters have to be changed every two to three days to prevent phlebitis and infection. If you suspect that you will be in and out of a drowsy state as you recuperate, let your friend or family member know that these are things to watch out for, and let them be your eyes while yours are resting
- Ask your physician daily if the intravenous line or catheter is still necessary. The longer they stay in, the greater the odds of getting an infection.

- Urinary catheters can and should be hooked up to triple lumen catheters, which allow sterile liquids to irrigate your bladder continually.
- When urinary catheters are removed, the nurse should first insert a few ounces of 0.25 percent solution acidic acid into your bladder to kill off the bacteria that will remain behind.
- Preoperative patients should be shaved with a clipper and not a razor. Abraded and scratched skin can become infected more easily.
- Do not accept an antibiotic unless the wound, urine, or blood was adequately cultured. You do not want to take the wrong antibiotic, which could mask the real culprit.
- As with outpatient procedures, get your surgery done first thing in the morning. The operating room is presumed to be the most sterile and not yet contaminated by a previous case. The surgeon and operating team are bright-eyed and bushy-tailed. I reviewed a case where a patient was the second one of the day to have a dilation and curettage (D&C) for a stillborn. The first patient had had a similar procedure done, but she also had hepatitis C. Unfortunately, the second patient came down with the same strain of hepatitis C six weeks later.
- Call the hospital's quality control, risk management, or infection control nurse and get the infection statistics for your physician as compared to his or her peers as well as the general risk compared to other hospitals.
- Check out the hospital on Web sites that compare hospitals' national averages.[17]
- Medical workers favor institutions that attract nurses. The American Nurses Association's Web site lists "magnet hospitals," those most attractive to nurses.
- Call the hospital's nursing supervisor and find out the nurse-to-patient ratio.

14

MEDICAL TESTS AND HOW TO AVOID BECOMING A LAB RAT!

Treat the patient, not the X-ray.

—James M. Hunter[1]

During the Yom Kippur war between Israel and the surrounding Arab states, I was working in the region as a volunteer physician. Because of my specialty in infectious diseases, I was asked to figure out why there were so many unusual infections on those wounded during combat. After reviewing a few hundred patient records, the answer became obvious. Everyone who was removed from the front lines was given multiple doses of various antibiotics. Then, when the helicopters flew the wounded to the rear-line hospitals, they were again given antibiotics. The unusual bacteria that remained alive were allowed to multiply, causing the unusual infections. The ironic part of this episode was the order for all combatants who were removed from the field to receive antibiotics, regardless of their ailment. This included a dozen soldiers who suffered from kidney stones as a result of the desert heat and dehydration and some soldiers who were shell shocked. In other words, it was a blanket treatment that did not pertain to everyone, and the medical staff just followed orders without thinking twice.

The interesting thing is that this experience is not unique to the military or the battlefield. This is, in fact, what happens every day with medical tests and prescription drugs. Practitioners are prescribing and patients are taking antibiotics without a whole lot of thinking. The result of this autopilot routine is that those jumbo jets are crashing and killing, or injuring, too many of the patients onboard.

Being a good patient and following my advice, after Doris was sent for an MRI of her chest, she requested that a copy of the results be sent to her. She called to let me know that her mammogram was normal and the lump I was suspicious of was therefore nothing to be concerned about. I called the radiology department to inform them that I did not order a mammogram for Doris, but an MRI. What was the problem? After researching the matter, the head technician called and apologized. "Everyone who is seen on Thursday afternoons is scheduled for a mammogram," she explained. Because there was no addended report, the receptionist assumed that (a) Doris had a mammogram done and (b) it must have been read as normal. The MRI, the test that was really done, proved *abnormal*. Try explaining that to the patient. And what if I hadn't called to check on it? There would have been no follow-up, no further treatment. Just more autopilot, sending patients crashing and burning.

Make sure that the test you are there for is the test you need. Make sure you get a copy of your results. That also means that they must have your proper address and phone number. While you are at it, make sure your personal physician's name and contact information are there and correct. There are many times that we receive the report of another physician's patient, in error. We then have to contact the lab or radiological facility for them to send the results to the correct physician. That is lots of time lost when time can be of utmost importance.

RADIOLOGY

The role of a radiologist is to recognize an abnormality, accurately diagnose it, and communicate the results to the patient and the physician. Imagine you are a woman over 40 years of age and it is time for your mammogram. No problem. I simply give you a prescription and you are off. Right? Wrong. One out of three mammograms will be mistakenly read. That is, one cancer out of three will be misread as normal. Furthermore, many palpable lumps may never show up on a mammogram. Any lump found must be evaluated with a mammogram, an ultrasound, and, ultimately, by an expert breast surgeon. Going to your internist or obstetrician/gynecologist would be a start to obtain the above testing, but in this day and age, the patient must follow up with a breast specialist. Delay in the diagnosis of breast cancer is the most common reason for malpractice lawsuits in the United States and, even more importantly, the proper treatment of the disease.[2] By now you probably know what I am going to say, but just in case: don't expect your physician or radiologist to be checking and double checking these things. Take it upon yourself to make sure you get the right test, accurate results, and the necessary follow ups.

Twelve percent of radiology-related medication errors, including incorrect dosing of sedatives or contrast agents, result in harm to the patient.[3] That is seven times the percentage of all medication errors combined that were harmful. What does this mean to you? It means that your questioning does not stop with your primary doctor. You must continue to question the lab technicians and radiologist. Do not be afraid to make a casual mention that you have read how many errors are made in incorrect dosing of sedatives and contrast agents, and that you are a little concerned about that needle they are about to put in your arm! Do you think they might stop and think twice about that routine procedure that they are about to perform on you? I think the odds are good they will.

Years ago, my dad had some mild midback pain. Having had heart disease in the past, I became overly cautious and sent him to the local radiologist. I did not think there was anything wrong, but I asked the doctor to check my dad out for an aortic aneurysm. A few hours later, the radiologist called me to let me know all was well. Two to three days later, my brother called from a hospital emergency room. "Dad was brought in with back pain and died almost immediately." The death sounded like a ruptured aneurysm, as the cardiac workup was negative. We chose not to do an autopsy. I called my local radiologist and presented the scenario of the night before. I asked him to review the x-rays he had done on my dad—not to be litigious but to learn if my brother or I had to be concerned for a future aneurysm. He called back and said, "Funny, we can't seem to find that x-ray."

The next year, my first wife awoke one morning with a hard lymph node in her left supraclavicular area (above her clavicle). I immediately sent her to another local radiologist for a mammogram and chest x-ray. Breast cancer and lung cancer are the two prime suspects in supraclavicular lymph node enlargements. I was called and told all was okay. Susan made an appointment with her internist the following week and was hospitalized for a complete workup. Another chest x-ray was done that showed the cause of her lymph node enlargement: lung cancer. It was only one week apart and would have been completely missed if another film had not been done.

Susan always had an annual chest x-ray done. For some reason, she skipped the previous year. Looking at the x-ray from two years ago, one could see a tiny, tiny spot where the cancer of today was found. Had she taken her annual x-ray the year before, I am sure her lung cancer would have been detected in time for a cure. Sadly, it was not. Survival of a disease is dependent upon early detection. This is why I believe in annual chest x-rays even though insurance carriers do not find them cost-effective.

Clearly, I am not hiding the fact that my loved ones have been victims of, if not malpractice, less than conscientious health care practices. And I would not hide the fact that these experiences are, in some part, my motivation for wanting to change the way this system works. But the truth is, besides my family members, I have seen examples like this—and far worse—perpetrated on far too many people (as I have described throughout this book). But most importantly, I am sharing these personal experiences to drive home the fact that, if these things can happen to the loved ones of a trained physician, they can happen to anyone if they do not take an active part in their health care decisions. Radiologists are presented with an enormous volume of x-rays and have to keep up with the newest and latest technologies. In order not to fall victim to errors, we must stand firm and demand to know as much as there is to know about every procedure offered. We have to have the conviction to demand second reads and of making sure that our tests are properly labeled. Only by taking responsibility for our health will we help avoid errors in our care.

LABORATORIES

No one really knows how many laboratory errors happen annually. A typical large medical center does some 5 million tests annually.[4] The testing starts in the doctor's office. Either your blood, urine, or biopsy specimen is obtained there, or a prescription is given from your physician for the tests to be obtained at an outside laboratory. Specimens are drawn and labeled. They are then sent to the specialized department (hematology, chemistry, or another expert) to be analyzed and interpreted. The results are then sent back to the doctor. Errors can occur anywhere in this pipeline, which can potentially threaten one's health or life. The most common laboratory error is that of mislabeling, or putting incorrect patient or doctor data on the laboratory specimen. If the wrong doctor is entered, it may fatally delay an abnormal result getting to the right physician in time.

Almost 3 million lab identification errors occur annually in the United States. Of that group, over 160,000 patients are harmed in some way.[5] Imagine the stress and anxiety that one experiences when given a terrible diagnosis, only later to discover that it was incorrect. Worse, of course, is to be given a normal diagnosis, leading to no further follow up or treatment, only to find out the results were abnormal and it is now too late for treatment. As an intern, I remember being part of a code (cardiopulmonary resuscitation) on a patient. Unfortunately, the patient could not be resuscitated and expired, as they say in medical vernacular. Let's call it what it was—the patient died. In the same way that politicians and the military use nicer sounding phrases to describe the carnage they wreak, like "collateral damage," "Operation Freedom," and so on, medical practitioners too are often guilty of hiding behind their own form of medical spin. The charge nurse told me that the family was in the waiting room. So off I went to inform the family of the patient's demise. This was my first encounter as a physician with a family who had lost someone. After giving them the bad news and experiencing their grief, I returned to the nurse's station to learn that I had told the wrong family! Fortunately, when they were told the good news, they were too relieved to be too upset. Personally, I wouldn't have blamed them for wanting to throw a punch my way.

I once employed a physician's assistant who ran a blood test on a patient and found the white blood cell count to be 50,000, which is very, very high (normal is up to 10,000). Instead of following the policy of repeating a bad, unexpected laboratory result, he went and told the patient that he had leukemia. Ten minutes later, the proper result came out of the machine and, again, there was a tremendous sigh of relief from the family of the patient who thought that he was going to die. One can only imagine how a family would have to deal with this diagnosis if they were not told the truth for a week or two.

Similarly, one could receive the wrong blood transfusion because of a mistake in labeling of one's blood type. One could also have a delay in treatment because someone else received your diagnosis. There are patients who undergo surgery unnecessarily because of the wrong diagnosis due to identification error. You know the old anecdote where the guy gets the wrong leg amputated. The doctor calls his lawyer and exclaims, "I just cut the wrong leg off my patient!" To which the lawyer calmly responds, "Don't worry, he can't sue you. He doesn't have a leg to stand on." Unfortunately, this is not an urban legend.

There are approximately 305,000 pathology specimens wrongly diagnosed each year, and 128,000 (40 percent) of those misdiagnosed pathology specimens will result in harm.[6] Laboratories should institute double checks on all their specimens. Hospitals should ensure that surgeons doing biopsies send properly diagnosable tissue samples to the pathology laboratory. At every step of the way, there is the possibility of misinformation, misdiagnoses, mislabeling, and the resulting medical errors that follow. Again this is not meant to scare you, but to make you aware of the realities of the medical world. Only then can you traverse the medical minefield without stepping on one of these mines.

So what do you do in these situations? If you are under sedation, you are obviously not going to be able to lean over and remind your doctor to get a good biopsy and make sure your name is written correctly on the sample being sent off to the lab. And you are most likely not going to pay a visit to the actual lab and follow the footprints of your sample to make sure it is correctly labeled and tested all along the way. But again, what you can do is alert your doctor, surgeon, or nurse to your concerns. Ask them to please double check that they have the right sample, a good sample, and the correct labeling. Then ask to see the actual sample to make sure for yourself that it is labeled correctly. For example, when you are getting your blood taken or giving a urine sample, take a moment to check the labels they are pasting on the jar or tube. After a biopsy, ask to see the sample so you can double check that the information is correct. If you get an abnormal result back, ask to have it checked again—and consider getting a second opinion. If you get a normal result back, go over it with your doctor and talk about whether or not there is any possibility that this result could be a false negative. Incidentally, most radiologists that I know ask for two readings when it comes to their own families. Furthermore, if the two physicians are part of the same radiology practice, they cannot charge twice for reading the same x-ray. It is against the law.

As you can see, many of these things are starting to sound familiar. While there are a few new specifics with each experience, overall it is about implementing the same basic proactive procedures before, during, and after tests and treatments. It is about shifting your mindset, then learning a set of new skills that will better prepare you to ask the right questions, ask enough questions, and demand sufficient answers. These new skills will allow you to relate to your medical practitioners in a kind, personable, but firm manner, and follow through until you are truly satisfied with your results.

PRESCRIPTION

Radiology

- We must, politely, insist that x-rays, scans, MRIs, ultrasounds, and CT scans be read by two radiologists. I understand that this may go against some doctors' protocol, but if you have your primary doctor request this, the radiologist will usually comply.
- Obtain copies of all your x-rays or scans. If your physician asks for the copies, they will usually be sent free of charge.
- Get two separate readings for mammograms. Mammograms are best obtained from centers that do hundreds, or thousands, a week, rather than just a few. To increase the accuracy of the readings, find a center where the reader also does the biopsies of the breast for abnormal mammograms. Most breast biopsies are now done by radiologists, and these reader/biopsy specialists, because of their experience, tend to give the most accurate readings.
- X-rays have to be properly labeled with the proper name, right and left sides identified. Whether done in a physician's office, at the local radiologist, or at the hospital, be nosey and ask to see the proper labeling. This may be intimidating to a patient to ask for these details, but if you are polite and humble and honestly express your concern about improper labeling based on your research, most medical practitioners will oblige. If they do not, you can still demand it—and they must provide it.
- Getting dye studies at the hospital or local radiologist office can be dangerous or even deadly. Make sure you inform the radiologist of all of your allergies and your concerns. Especially let them know if you are a diabetic and if you are taking other medicines.
- If you are a smoker (goodness knows why), or are an ex-smoker, you should definitely get a baseline spiral CT scan of your lungs. Thousands

of patients have tiny lung cancers that can be picked up while the cancer is in its infancy and in its curable stage.

- Ask if this procedure is really necessary and if there is a safer procedure.
- Keep copies of all of your x-rays and their corresponding reports.
- Go over the reports with your physician and make sure everything is explained to your satisfaction.

Lab Work

- Ask your physician or surgeon to order the laboratory to have multiple pathologists examine pathology slides or Pap tests. This will lessen the chance that cancer cells go undetected.
- If you have questions about laboratory results, diagnosis, or treatments, speak up and be persistent.
- Call for results of tests. Do not assume that if the doctor didn't call you all is fine. There are times that I do not receive the blood results and therefore do not know whether my patients have normal or abnormal tests.
- Do not worry about hurting your doctor's feelings, after he reads this book he will agree with whatever you ask.
- Read your laboratory identification slip or sticker when your blood is sent out of your physician's office or a laboratory, making sure that your name and your physician's name are correct. Be as diligent as if you were reviewing a bill at an expensive restaurant.
- If a laboratory result is unexpectedly abnormal (or for that matter normal) or alarming, make sure you have it repeated. Remember, radiologists have their own family members get two readings.
- Keep copies of all laboratory tests and biopsy reports.

⑮

MAJOR SURGERIES: OR HOW TO MAKE SURE YOU STILL HAVE A LEG TO STAND ON AFTERWARD!

I got the bill for my surgery. Now I know what those doctors were wearing masks for.

—James H. Boren[1]

Things You Don't Want to Hear in the Operating Room

- Don't worry, I think it's sharp enough.
- Nurse, did this patient sign the organs donation card?
- Page 84 of the manual is missing!
- Everybody stand back, I lost a contact lens!
- Oops.
- Better save that, we'll need it for the autopsy.
- Wait a minute, if this is the spleen, then what's that?
- What do you mean "you want a divorce"?

Being athletically active, I have become more prone to surgical orthopedic procedures. I have had cartilage in both knees removed and had torn rotator cuffs repaired in both shoulders. With each injury came the agonizing choice of "to cut or not to cut." There is the apprehension (my fear) of needing general anesthesia. Will I wake up or become comatose? Will I suffer a lot of postoperative pain and disability? Can I live with the injury and just limit the activities to those I now can do? Will I develop a wound infection that could possibly ruin my joint forever? Will I succumb to a fat or blood embolism and wake up on a respirator? My choice for surgery has always been to maintain the quality of life that I enjoy. Bicycling, working out, practicing tae kwon do, playing tennis, and, of course, taking long walks (especially on vacation) have always pushed my envelope to have surgery. So the fun often trumps the fear.

When it comes to the operating room, I have the same fears and anxieties common to all of us. My presurgical blood pressure shoots sky high and my pulse races up to the nineties (usually I am 120/80 with a pulse of 60, which is considered normal). After signing a multitude of consent forms and having an intravenous line started, I start to shiver a little. The ride on the gurney through the operating room, passing all the operating suites, is always fun, especially when the surgeons and nurses who are friends, point their thumbs up for good luck. Then they put you on the table, or you are actually encouraged to shimmy off the gurney unto the operating room table, without exposing your private parts (always a tough assignment, because of the loose and untied hospital gown). Then there is the washing, scrubbing, and possible shaving—downright humiliating, especially if you know everyone. Then you really start shivering, and it is not from fear. Operating rooms are kept at freezing temperatures, ostensibly to keep the bacteria in the air from multiplying and causing infections. (We all know infections will happen to some of us, but hopefully all that shivering and shaking will bounce the bacteria into another room!) Next comes the taping of your arms and intravenous line to the side board, while nurses throw hot blankets over you to keep you warm. Then the anesthesiologist is ready, and by the time you can count to three, the lights are out.

Unlike the television show *ER*, people are not rushed from the emergency room to the operating room. There are very few instances where immediate emergency surgery is necessary within minutes or an hour. Massive bleeding (due to a motor vehicle accident, gun shot, or stabbing wounds) is one such emergency. However, more likely scenarios involve slow bleeding, especially from ruptured abdominal organs. This allows for the interplay of various specialties (gastroenterologists, surgeons) and the use of CT and MRI. These will help localize the source of blood loss, thereby more effectively leading the surgeon to the affected site. This gap in time will also give the patient and his or her family a chance to decide whether surgery should be done emergently, or at all. Remember earlier in the book I mentioned the case of one hospital when more surgeons started working in that hospital, and magically more surgeries were performed. Keep that in mind. The hungrier the surgeon, the quicker he or she will want to jump in right away. I say let him or her stay hungry—let him or her starve—if that is what it takes to make the right decision. And that is exactly what you must do, make the *right* decision; a decision that is informed not by fear, panic, or pressure from doctors and, in some cases, even loved ones. If you are conscious and coherent, take the time to ask lots of questions:

- Do I really need surgery?
- Is this the best type of surgery to perform for this condition, or are there less-invasive alternatives (laparoscopy, local anesthesia, etc.)?
- What are the possible side effects or drug interactions with whatever medications and anesthesia that will be given?
- Is there another doctor who can give me a second opinion—either on the labs/test/x-rays or on the diagnosis and surgery itself?
- Can I have a loved one or patient's advocate observe the procedure?
- Can I wait until morning to have the surgery? (Remember, the operating room first thing in the morning is the most sanitary, and the doctors are usually the most alert.)
- Can I get a laptop with Internet and do some Googling?! (You may not get this one but, hey, it doesn't hurt to ask!)

The most common scenario, however, involves presenting to your physician, who will do a series of tests and determine that you have an elective surgical event. Now the decision making is purely yours. Now you have time for due diligence. Almost daily, we identify patients with gallstones, kidney stones, lumps in their breasts, growths on their ovaries, or uterine tumors. It is good to have a fear of surgery and its complications, so that you do not rush into things. And it is good to have some time to investigate your problem and think it over. But if there is a real medical problem, intelligent and educated decisions must still be made in a timely fashion. Second opinions are certainly very important and, in fact, some insurance companies require them. Other questions to ask (which you could also ask in the above scenario, although you may not have the choice as to which surgeon you use):

- Are there alternatives?
- Can the disease be controlled medically?
- What are the odds of survival?
- What qualities does my surgeon possess that are beneficial?

- How many procedures does he or she do annually?
- What's his or her success rate? Infection rate? Complication rate?

These are questions most of us are faced with at some point in our lives. For these answers, we need a concerned internist, the Internet, a qualified surgeon, and, of course, a hospital that has sworn and proven to protect its patients from harm. We know that studies show the vast amount of injuries are caused within hospitals themselves, but studies also show that more patients are injured by their hospital and its employees than by general surgeons. As I mentioned earlier, hospital statistics are available for infection rates, complication rates, and so on. HealthGrades Web site provides information on both your hospital and your physician. The National Department of Health Web site offers "Hospital Compare" and other databases that measure the overall quality of care for all hospitals. "Hospital Compare" especially details care for heart failure, heart attacks, pneumonia, and surgical care. Use these sites and tools to make sure your hospital of choice is a safe one.

PRIOR TO SURGERY

Most states have developed testing and guidelines for patients prior to undergoing surgery. Electrocardiograms, x-rays, special blood testing (especially to ensure that the patient's blood will not be too thin), and a thorough physical examination are routine. The physical examination, aside from ensuring that the heart and other organs can withstand surgery, is also important for localizing any preexisting infection. It is obvious that if your head is clogged with a cold or sinus inflammation, breathing during or after surgery would be difficult. Less obvious, however, is a skin infection even remotely away from the surgical site. If you have a boil or infected area of your back and you are having leg surgery, for example, there will be a higher chance of getting a wound infection with the same bacteria.

I remember one patient who developed *herpes zoster* (shingles) the day before surgery. Unyielding, the surgeon wanted to perform the elective gallbladder removal, as scheduled, despite my concern that the patient could have spread her localized viral infection. In this case, the infection did not spread. *But it easily could have.* This was much more about schedules and egos than it was about the ultimate safety and well-being of the patient. And this happens every day. Just because the patient was okay with it does not justify this type of practice. That is like someone saying that just because they haven't gotten into a car accident yet while talking on their cell phone and putting on makeup on the way to work, it is a perfectly safe way to travel. But that, unfortunately, is the mentality that sometimes runs our decisions—in our private lives as well as the medical profession.

ANTIBIOTICS AND DRUG INTERACTION
BEFORE SURGERY

Many patients are placed on antibiotics for an infection the week, or perhaps days, prior to the day of surgery. These antibiotics just change the flora (the types) of bacteria on the skin to another group of bacteria, *they do not sterilize the skin*. If an infection occurs, because of the use of these kinds of antibiotics, it would be more difficult to guess which bacteria are causing the infection. As discussed earlier, this can lead to a misdiagnosis of the underlying bacteria and the wrong treatment, which can lead to serious complications. Many times the surgeon is not made aware of the fact that his or her patient was treated for some other infection, with an antibiotic, prior to performing surgery. The patient may have seen a dentist for a tooth abscess and been placed on an antibiotic. The patient may have seen her private physician or gynecologist for a urinary tract infection. The consequences of being on an antibiotic that changes the types of bacteria on the skin can be very serious. Solution: *You must notify your surgeon if you were on an antibiotic prior to surgery. Better still, notify your internist.*

Many complications, during and postoperatively, occur in patients who are on long-term cortisone therapy. These patients include those who suffer with asthma, collagen disease, and severe allergies. Oral cortisone suppresses the body's ability to rapidly produce steroids on their own. Either not knowing that the patient was on cortisone or not realizing the consequences has caused many complications. Steroids are produced by the body at the moment of stress. They are made to maintain a good, strong blood pressure. Patients, whose response to stress is suppressed because they have been taking cortisone therapy, will go into shock unless they are given higher doses of cortisone prior to their surgery. Surgery is a tremendous shock to the body, which requires the body to respond by producing high doses of cortisone. If one takes cortisone therapy regularly, they will have an inability to produce their own cortisone. The extra cortisone has to be supplemented by the physician.

Make sure that you discuss all of the medications you are taking with your internist and surgeon prior to your surgery. Make sure you know the consequences of what will happen to you if you do or do not take the medicines prior to surgery. My mother did not take her blood pressure medicines prior to her having carotid artery surgery. The surgeon had to wait an hour after administering his own batch of blood pressure lowering medicines before he performed her surgery.

The "new" male has become an enormous consumer of sildenafil (Viagra) and related sexually stimulating medications. Your anesthesiologist must know if you have any of that type of medication in your system. Certain medications used during surgery (which includes nitroglycerin if your blood pressure rises) could have a deleterious effect on those using this type of medication. Many patients are too embarrassed, or unknowing, to relate their use of these drugs to the hospital staff. Don't be one of them.

The fact is, many patients are on a multitude of medications and can become confused about which to take and which not to take the morning of surgery. If you take any medications, make sure to discuss which ones you should take with your doctor prior to surgery. And then arrange, in advance, a telephone conversation with the anesthesiologist the day before surgery to confirm which medications you can take (as a general rule, all cardiac and blood pressure medications should be taken) the morning of surgery. Because you might be a little nervous about the procedure, make sure to write out your questions in advance of the doctor appointment and the phone call with the anesthesiologist. If you feel the need for additional support, it also wouldn't hurt to have a friend or loved one look over your list to make sure you have written all the medications and questions down, and then to be by your side to make sure you cover everything with your physician and anesthesiologist. Having surgery is not something you do every day (at least I hope not!). So don't take it lightly. And don't hesitate to call on friends, loved ones, and your primary doctor to go the extra mile during this time.

PROPHYLACTIC ANTIBIOTICS

Prophylactic antibiotics is a term used for administrating antibiotics in a large enough amount to patients who are susceptible to infection. It is like a contraceptive to prevent the bacteria from ever getting in (or at least from taking hold in the system), or a birth control pill versus the "morning after" pill. In surgical parlance, prophylactic antibiotics are generally given to patients with artificial heart valves, or those who have internal "hardware," such as artificial joints or metal rods, plates, and so on. These areas of damage (heart valves), or inanimate metallic objects, have no blood supply. The concept is that when bacteria enter the bloodstream during surgery, the antibiotics immediately kill them off. The antibiotics are usually given one to two hours prior to surgery through the intravenous line. This is to attain the highest antibiotic level in the bloodstream, as well as to keep the patient fasting. The concept behind giving the antibiotic one to two hours prior to surgery is to give enough antibiotics to intercept the most common organisms that are going to get into the bloodstream. If surgery is going to be through the skin (as opposed to the mouth), the most common organism expected to get into the blood and cause infection is staphylococcus. If one were having surgery in the mouth or rectum, other organisms would be involved.

Many patients fail to tell their surgeons that they have artificial valves or that there is a metal plate or other artificial object in their body. In other words, oftentimes the patient is complicit in his or her own malpractice. By not offering full disclosure—out of fear, guilt, pride, or shame—the patient is setting him- or herself on a course of further complications. Of course, as doctors it is our responsibility to ask the right questions that draw out these important discoveries. Nevertheless, this shows just how important it is that you, the patient, play your part in your medical procedures. Tell your doctor *everything* that may be pertinent—and even that which may not be. At the very worst, you will just bore your doctor with useless information (if you do see his or her face start to glaze over, however, you might want to shift your tactics). More often, however, you will be giving your doctor a clearer picture to work from.

One of my patients recently had hair transplantation, and the scalp, being composed of skin, is laden with staphylococci. The topnotch plastic surgeon he went to gave my patient a prescription for one week of antistaphylococcus medication. I tried explaining to the surgeon that by the time of surgery, he would have killed off all of the susceptible staphylococci. However, the area would be recolonized by different bacteria, which would not be susceptible to this antibiotic. One cannot sterilize the skin by oral or intravenous antibiotics. Other bacteria, present from the beginning in minuscule amounts, would start to grow in leaps and bounds when the staphylococci (which was keeping their growth in check) were killed off. This is called recolonization. One of these newly emerged bacteria would then be involved in an infection he was originally trying to prevent. (At the risk of drawing too broad a metaphor here, it is sort of like the problems with Iraq post-9/11. When Saddam was in power, as bad as he was, he kept the many other potentially feuding forces in check. The minute he was "killed off," however, these heretofore relatively benign forces grew out of control until they had recolonized the country and created a much worse problem than before.)

There is only one preparation, which can be purchased over the counter, that has been proven to prevent postantibiotic usage diarrhea,[2] that is, if the diarrhea is not specifically caused by *Clostridium difficile*. This probiotic, *Saccharomyces boulardii* (Florastor), has also been used to prevent travelers' diarrhea and is used as a treatment for diarrhea in general. The pill should be taken daily while on antibiotics and started a few days before prophylactic antibiotics are given. To prevent travelers' diarrhea, it should also be taken daily, but started a few days before travel.[3]

ANTICOAGULATION THERAPY

Anticoagulation therapy in the preoperative patient is an important matter to discuss for those with artificial heart valves, abnormal heart rhythms, and a host of other preclotting conditions. Anticoagulation therapy involves thinning of the blood so that clots do not form. Patients are usually on warfarin (Coumadin) for the above reasons. If not, clots would form on the surface of their heart valve and be shot off into their brains as an embolism.

The problem is you do not want your blood too thin when you are going to have surgery. You want clots to form or you could bleed to death. No surgeon wants to cut into a patient who is not going to stop bleeding. (No patient wants that either, I might add.) Patients are usually asked to stop their anticoagulation medication five days before surgery. The reasoning is that the patient would only be at risk for getting a clot for a few days, as the warfarin gradually wears off. This is certainly better than bleeding to death. But it also poses risks. A dangerous clot can still form. So there are alternatives. Short-term (twelve-hour) injectable therapy has been around for a few years. These are anticoagulants that are injected into the skin, given every twelve hours, and stopped the morning of surgery. Therefore, the risk of clotting is minimized to only the morning of surgery, and the therapy is restarted that same evening. Continued injections are given for the next week, the time that is takes for the warfarin to kick in.

Many patients or their families are nervous at the thought of injecting themselves. You know what I say to that by now—*get over it!* Many patients, however, are never even offered this potentially life-saving option. You, the proactive patient, should know your risk of clotting and what preventative measures are available to you. Many a patient has suffered from a brain clot because of not being adequately anticoagulated during the perisurgical period (that time encompassing days before and days after the actual surgery). A well-known case is former president Richard Nixon, who suffered from atrial fibrillation. It has been strongly suggested that he died of a brain embolism because his anticoagulation therapy for this cardiac arrhythmia was not restarted in a timely fashion after he had gallbladder surgery.

PRESCRIPTION

Preoperative

- Talk to your primary doctor and surgeon in depth about the surgical procedure and make sure to get all your questions and concerns dealt with (if it is an emergency, you may not have as much time for this, but if you are conscious and coherent, ask questions).
- Research on your own about the surgery, the complications, and the possible alternatives—and discuss your concerns with your doctor and surgeon, as well as possibly getting a second opinion.
- Make sure your doctor, surgeon, and anesthesiologist know the medications you are taking, and schedule a call with the anesthesiologist the day before surgery to confirm which medications you should or should not take the morning of surgery.
- If at all possible, schedule your surgery first thing in the morning.
- Make sure to disclose all preexisting conditions (artificial heart valves, internal hardware, etc.) and talk about prophylactic antibiotics to prevent infection.
- If you are on any kind of anticoagulant—for cardiac arrhythmias or other issues—make sure your surgeon knows about it and the proper

steps are taken to either stop the medication several days before surgery or take the daily injections (as described above).

- Observe everything around you. I recently had minor surgery on my finger and the anesthesiologist became so chatty that, after starting my intravenous line, she forgot to turn on the solution. As she walked away I reminded her. The intravenous line is there as an emergency lifeline, in case one needs life-saving medication. It would not have done me any good had the needle clogged without the solution running through it.
- If you have a particular music that soothes you, ask to have it played in the operating room, and ask that your surgeons and other medical practitioners refrain from negative or unrelated talk (studies have shown that conversations during surgery have adversely affected patients even while being anesthetized).
- If possible, have a patient's advocate, friend, or family member close by at all times before, during, and after surgery.

Postoperative

- Do not be afraid to move or breathe deeply. There will be pain and the wound will feel as if it is going to tear apart. It won't. And the sutures will not pop out. It is just the pressure that you feel because the sutures are pulling the muscles together.
- Get out of bed as soon as you can and stay out as much as you can.
- Wear pressure stockings to keep the circulation going in your legs. Poor venous circulation in the lower extremities, from not moving or lying in bed for prolonged periods, can lead to thrombosis (clotting of a vein) of the veins and possibly a pulmonary embolism (clot).
- If you had a surgical procedure or one done by a surgical subspecialist (urologist, orthopedist) and you develop a complication, do not be treated by the house doctor but by the same specialist. I am testifying against a house doctor who tried to insert a urinary catheter into the bladder of a patient who had just undergone radical prostate surgery. The catheter either fell out or was pulled out by the semiconscious patient and the on-call urologist did not want to go in to see the patient and asked the house physician to take care of it. After such a complicated operation, only a urologist, using a cystoscope, is trained to do the catheter placement. This patient has suffered so many

complications because of the laziness or misjudgement of the on-call urologist.

- Try to get your catheter and intravenous line out as soon as possible (to limit risk of infection). The longer that they remain in you, the risk of infection increases greatly.
- Try to avoid the use or dependence on narcotics or pain medication. That is not to say that you should not take pain medicine if you are truly in pain. Too often patients rely on these drugs for minor pain and the consequences can ensue rapidly. Narcotics cause constipation and more importantly, dependence. Opium was used widely for the treatment of diarrhea years ago because of its constipating effect, but no one wants to suffer from constipation after an abdominal operation.

IV

THE FUTURE OF MEDICINE

16

A CURE FOR THE MEDICAL SYSTEM

Fixing our healthcare system as a whole is our primary challenge, and to make it happen you need to get engaged—to pound the pavement, get your hands dirty, endure real sacrifice, take on antiquated thinking and help lead the public debate.

—Senator John Kerry[1]

On the national political side, we have to acknowledge the fact that our health care system is broken. Over 45 million Americans have no health care coverage at all. Another 40 million citizens have only minimal coverage. Furthermore, an additional 40 percent of moderate and middle-income Americans go without insurance for part of the year. Over 50 percent of people earning $20,000 annually have no insurance at all. It is estimated that 18,000 people in the United States die every year because of a lack of health insurance.[2] The World Health Organization (WHO) ranks the United States thirty-seventh in the world for health system performance. Yes, contrary to the popular myth perpetrated by many politicians, we do *not* have the best health care system in the world. Far from it. If that isn't enough, the citizens of thirty-five other nations live longer than we do.

According to a January 10, 2008, article in the *Journal News*, the United States placed last among nineteen industrialized countries in a study comparing preventable deaths. (This article summarized a report from The

Commonwealth Fund.) Although advances in medical science have offered patients and health care professionals life-saving techniques, tools, and treatments unavailable in the past, according to the report, "by many measures the U.S. health care system isn't performing as well as it could." The United States had the highest infant mortality rate and tied with New Zealand and the United Kingdom for the lowest average healthy life expectancy. Most amazingly, those in the United States pay the most money, per capita, and yet still receive such inferior health care. The United States spends more than any other industrialized nation—more than $2 trillion, or $7,026 per citizen—yet cannot deliver health care to everyone who needs it. This was according to The Commonwealth Fund, a private foundation that promotes health care reform. Just eight years ago, in 2000, we spent almost half, $1.4 trillion for our health care. There is so much variability from state to state and city to city, as well as hospital to hospital, in the health care provided by doctors and hospitals that if all states performed as well as Minnesota, an estimated 90,000 premature deaths could be prevented each year.[3]

Unfortunately, child health care varies widely among the states. In a nationwide report compiled by The Commonwealth Fund, only 46 percent of children visit the doctor or dentist at least once a year in Idaho, but 75 percent of Massachusetts's children do. Infant mortality rates are 2.5 times higher in the District of Columbia than in Maine. Interestingly, the District of Columbia has the highest spending per person for health care in the nation, $8,295, and is ranked thirty-first out of the fifty states and the District of Columbia. Utah has the lowest spending per person, at $3,972, and is ranked twenty-sixth, quite a difference in dollars but not much of a difference in ranking.

The Fund analyzed thirteen measures of children's care, including access, quality, and costs for each state. Top performing states have lower rates of uninsured than those ranked at the bottom. But they have higher health costs.

The percentage of American children who received five recommended vaccinations varied widely from 94 percent in Massachusetts to 67 percent in Nevada. Uninsured children ranged from 5.7 percent in Michigan to 20 percent in Texas. The conclusion of the study, which was reported in *USA Today*, May 5, 2008, was that if all states performed as well as the top states in each category:

1. an additional 4.6 million children nationwide would have health insurance;

2. 11.8 million more children would visit the doctor or dentist at least once a year;
3. 800,000 more children would be current with their vaccinations.[4]

Because of these variables in health care delivery, and the fact that insurance companies (and their HMOs) have taken over the practice of medicine, organized medicine has recently asked for some reform. It is interesting that the American Medical Association (AMA), with its proposal for reform, still wants the continued participation of the insurance companies in health care, whereas the American Medical Student Association sees the light and wants to part ways with insurance companies.[5] Senator Dennis Kucinich, democratic presidential primary challenger in the 2008 U.S. presidential election, called for universal health care. Following is a synopsis of the AMA's proposal, which deals mostly with obtaining health insurance for the uninsured:

- The AMA wants to pinpoint and address fundamental flaws in how people currently obtain and pay for health insurance, especially the flaws that limit the availability and affordability of coverage.
- Make better use of existing government resources devoted to health care and health care coverage, including the billions of dollars spent subsidizing employment-based private insurance with the wish to give these monies to people to pay for a health plan of their choosing.
- Expand health insurance coverage and improve fairness by shifting government spending toward those most likely to be uninsured.[6]

It is true that the uninsured are the largest group of victims of medical malpractice, but there was no mention of the problem of medical malpractice in this AMA proposal. There is no mention of fixing a dying system.

The fallout from the above statistics and the fact that U.S. physicians are working harder and harder just to match what they were making the year before is quite clear. Patients with little or no health insurance will continue to receive poor health care delivery. Busy, inattentive hospitals and physicians will try to cram more and more service into less and less hours, with limited or inadequate technology. I fear that they will make more mistakes and cause more malpractice injuries and deaths. And don't misunderstand my sympathy for doctors when I decry their struggle to make a living. I am not saying that doctors are two steps from the poorhouse. I am fully aware that they still rank above the average American in terms of pay. I must also acknowledge that they have, in most cases, earned this through a lot of hard work, a lot of lost sleep, and often a large student debt. The fact, however, is that they are human. And having accustomed themselves to the fruits of their labor, they, like most other humans, will continue to strive for those fruits. If the current system continues to reduce their pay, limit their effectiveness, overburden the staff and system with bureaucracy, raise malpractice insurance through the roof (despite the fact that a minority of doctors are responsible for the majority of medical errors), and then fail to take strong measures to discipline, retrain, or get rid of bad doctors, then the natural, albeit unfortunate, consequences will be the scenario I have described in this book—a scenario that is already in full swing.

Bottom line, the present system has to be overhauled and made more efficient and certainly more encompassing. The debate about universal health coverage by a single-payer system has been around for seventy years. It was swept under the carpet in the early 1990s with the introduction of insurance company–driven HMOs. This approach has also proven to be disastrous. Under a single-payer system, one government agency, Medicare, not hundreds of insurance companies, reimburses clinics and hospitals, and further sets limits on what clinics, hospitals, and drug companies can charge. High administrative costs generated by the current multiple-payer system would be reduced under a single-payer system. There are 1,500 insurance companies selling health care insurance. Each of these companies has their own hierarchy of administrators. The traditional Medicare program is more popular and more efficient than any insurance company. Medicare spends only 2 percent of its expenditures on overhead and spends the other 98 percent on health care. Conversely, insurance companies reward their administrators and spend a whopping 20 percent on overhead, leaving 80 percent to be returned to the health care system. What is more, insurance companies are in business to make a profit and are, in fact, obligated by law to deliver increased shareholder value. That means that they will do whatever it takes to reduce costs and increase revenues, even if it means reducing the quality and quantity of health care provided to their clients. It is nothing personal really, it is simple economics. It is also a vicious conflict of interest that, in the final analysis, cannot serve the people's needs best without radical reform.[7]

The money we are spending on health insurance is twice the amount spent by Canada and all of the other industrialized countries around the world.[8] All these other countries have universal health care systems. Under this new structure, health care will cost us less, be run more efficiently, and deliver better overall results. Certainly, Medicare cannot absorb the entire population in just one year. However, it can do so over a few years' time. Whether you agree with this particular approach or not, one thing is certain: the system we are using is not only failing, but will completely collapse unless we take measures to repair and remodel it.

Quoting Senator Kucinich: "We have the most expensive health care system in the world. We spend about twice as much per person as other developed nations, and that gap is growing. That's not because we are sicker or more demanding," as Canadians see their doctors more often and spend more time in the hospital than we do. "And it's not because we get better results. By the usual measures of health (life expectancy, infant mortality, immunization rates), we do worse than most other developed countries."[9] There is no question that the system is collapsing around us.

The intention of this book is to identify and acknowledge the existence of medical malpractice, which is an offshoot of this larger problem. This will, hopefully, enable the general public to protect themselves from this failing system. But I also hope to inspire action that will ultimately change the system from the inside out. In summary, there are multiple factors that are intertwined in this malpractice pandemic. One of the biggest issues is that most physicians do not accept the responsibility that malpractice occurs because of the following:

- Human nature (ego). A failure to admit that they could possibly have caused an error.
- Possible negative consequences of a bad "report card."
- Fear that their admittance will negate their contracts for coverage by the medical malpractice carrier.

MALPRACTICE INSURANCE AND FRIVOLOUS LAWSUITS

Although there are certainly doctors who deserve to be sued, and possibly have their licenses revoked, many physicians, especially surgeons, are sued for poor outcomes despite the fact that they did everything possible in their power to prevent and combat any complication. Because of our litigious society and the onslaught of real medical errors, doctors are often sued even when they truly did not make a preventable mistake. I was once asked to testify against an emergency room team that had saved a patient being admitted in cardiac arrest. During the drama and excitement of treatment, an intravenous line infiltrated (intravenous solutions leaking out of the vein and into the surrounding tissue), causing burning and, ultimately, scarring of the patient's upper arm. Yes, that was a poor outcome to the patient's arm and it arose from the intravenous team rushing to get that lifeline in. It was an error, in the literal sense, but it was based on the bigger urgency of acting quickly and saving a life. It was not medical malpractice. The patient's life was saved because of their quick and correct actions. In this case, that was the outcome that counted. Therefore, in this case, I did not testify for the plaintiff.

Hillary Rodham Clinton and Barack Obama coauthored an article in the prestigious *New England Journal of Medicine*: "Making Patient Safety the Centerpiece of Medical Liability Reform."[10] They understood the concerns and increased insurance financial burdens placed upon physicians. However, they also spoke with many families who suffered from medical malpractice and were empathetic with them. Therefore they summarized that the protection of the patient was the paramount goal.

It seems that medical malpractice insurance rates have been driven up recently because, until a few years ago, medical malpractice insurance companies lost money insuring physicians. The insurance companies made up for their losses by money made on other investments. Now they just want to make a profit, which, as mentioned earlier, is why they are in business. This does not mean this problem is unsolvable. But it does require that physicians take more responsibility. Here are the facts again:

- Physicians have to acknowledge that they make mistakes and that they are human.
- Patients deserve an apology because of an error and they should be compensated for their injuries.
- Malpractice occurs, it kills, and it costs society at least $36 billion annually.
- A small percentage of physicians are responsible for a very large percentage of these malpractice claims. These physicians are mostly not disciplined at all by the professional state agencies.

Many complaints by organized medicine ring true. The U.S. Department of Justice published malpractice trail data in the nation's seventy-five most populous counties. Of the 1,156 medical malpractice trials litigated, 90 percent involved plaintiffs (or their families) who claimed death or permanent injury. Approximately 25 percent of these plaintiffs won, 75 percent lost, suggesting a goodly number were frivolous, or as in many cases that I have participated in, the other side just had better lawyers.[11] To me, that is the most upsetting part. Malpractice insurance companies are also in the business to make money. They fight almost every case, whether the doctor was guilty or not. That is just not right. On the other hand, there are many frivolous cases. Frivolous cases suggest lawyers are more interested in making money rather than helping police a broken system. The amounts awarded to plaintiffs have been stable during these past ten years. In the seventy-five busiest counties, the total awards came to almost a half billion dollars. Furthermore, many studies show that increased malpractice insurance rates to doctors do not send specialists running out of their practices. Some may move to other "cheaper," less litigious counties. Most stay.

ORGANIZED MEDICINE, NOT LAWYERS, CAN FIGHT FOR PATIENTS' RIGHTS

Frivolous lawsuits (approximately 70 percent of all lawsuits) are wearing on physicians' time and money, as well as their practices. Too much time is spent in court and away from their patients. However, the conclusion of the study just cited above and published in the *New England Journal of Medicine* was that lack of evidence of malpractice is not uncommon and that most are denied compensation. The vast majority of expenditures go toward litigation over true medical malpractice and payments of them. The overhead costs of true medical practice are exorbitant. Until now, however, lawyers have been the only ones who have protected the rights of those who have been injured or killed. It has been suggested that $6 billion is spent annually for litigation of these cases. That figure represents legal fees on both sides but does not include awards.[12] If organized medicine wanted to intervene and protect patients' rights and, at the same time, lower the costs of malpractice, here is what they could offer:

- They could fight for a national data bank, reporting all errors.
- They could copy the work done by the American Society of Anesthesiology, which I reported earlier.

- They could accept responsibility for errors and malpractice.
- They could set up medical courts, governed by specialists in medical ethics and respected physicians.

The legal profession should still protect patients' rights. However, their fees should be lower and flat. The concept is to admit guilt and compensate the injured, not make fat cats out of anyone else. Reducing the amount of frivolous lawsuits would lower malpractice insurance rates, reduce barriers to admission by doctors in such cases, and increase overall rewards on legitimate cases. Similar to workers' compensation or disability awards, patients deserve fair compensation, which should be standardized.

Not to sound insensitive, but a loss of a limb is worth the same to everyone, whether it occurs in New York or Florida. The award should not be higher or lower because one person has a better lawyer than another or because the court is in a poorer neighborhood where higher awards may occur more frequently. The result of this kind of clarity and standardization would not be to lessen the rewards to patients but, ultimately, to increase them overall. I have observed that many lawyers now have to fight to prove that their clients were the victims of malpractice. That costs $6 billion annually. There would not be a fight if the physician were able and willing to admit guilt (i.e., if the insurance companies did not force them to be quiet at the risk of losing their insurance). The saving of the $6 billion, plus the savings of the 33 percent of awards that go to lawyers, would certainly lower the costs of medical malpractice insurance and thereby increase the overall coverage and rewards to those who deserve them.

These are just a few first steps toward lowering the legal and insurance costs until the medical profession gets its act together. A comprehensive approach involving the legal system, medicine, and the insurance companies needs to be undertaken. As it stands today, until medicine puts its house in order and reorganizes for the future, the health of our citizens will continue to suffer.

This week I received a case review. The wife of the plaintiff, Mary, wrote a summary of what she observed and has allowed me to print it:

July 06

John and I traveled to a cancer institute in upstate New York and a cancer clinic in New York City, for second and third opinions on whether the colostomy was necessary. Doctors at both of these institutions agreed with Dr. S, indicating that a colostomy was indeed needed.

Aug 06

John had a great deal of difficulty getting through the radiation and chemo-therapy. He was very much affected by it, ill and uncomfortable much of the time. The therapy sessions had to be halted and then resumed. His surgery was originally scheduled for November, about two weeks prior to Thanks-giving, but had to be postponed because it took him so long to get through the therapies. In retrospect, I wish we had postponed the surgery until after Christmas, because I believe that being near Christmas contributed to the neglect that he suffered while in the hospital.

Dec 06

We had a pre-operative discussion with Dr. S on what to expect from the surgery. No mention was made of the dangers of infection and sepsis in an operation of this sort, and it was portrayed as a rather routine procedure. I had to ask what complications we might expect, such as urinary or sexual difficulties, and was assured that complications were not often experienced, but could happen. Certainly, at this point, I wish that we had been given an education in infection control and the symptoms and signs of infection. I believe that hospital personnel and doctors and their staffs should undergo more rigorous education along these lines as well.

On December 8, John checked into the hospital for his surgery. Again, no mention was made of infection, neither in recognizing it nor controlling it. Having read about hospital based staph infections, I was appalled at how often I had to ask people to wash their hands before attending to John. And often they would just don gloves.

John had his surgery on December 8th, and besides being quite uncom-fortable initially, nothing seemed wrong. He seemed to get stronger and bet-ter every day. He was hooked up to an I.V. for fluids, he had a Foley catheter in, and a small plastic bottle attached to his side for the drainage of fluids in the abdomen. Eventually, they began to wean him off of these items, and introduced foods.

John's last good day was on December 13th. When I arrived, after work, he was sitting up in bed, no Foley, no little plastic bottle, reading the paper. The next day was a different story. On December 14th, when I went to visit, it was clear that he was in a good deal of discomfort again. The Foley was back in, as John said he wasn't able to urinate on his own but there was no little plastic bottle. He wasn't offered any fluids by mouth again, but I was told that his reaction was normal, that it takes time to get things going in the intestines. The next day, December 15th, the same thing, only John now said he was feeling more than just discomfort, that he was actually feeling sick. He was nauseous, and he felt like his heart was fluttering. I noticed that his urine output had slowed, almost stopped, and the color was dark, almost brown. The nurses said that was normal, that he was a little dehydrated. He was defecating into the colostomy bag, but it was of a very liquid nature, and smelled of sickness. I wanted this all reported to Dr. S but I was referred to an Intern, Dr. T, who cheerfully told me that all was well, that all these things were to be expected.

The next day or two, December 16th and 17th, were a bit of a blur. John continued to deteriorate, and the staff at the hospital and Dr. T continued to tell me that all was well and to be expected. John's heart rate was extremely elevated as was his respiration rate. His blood pressure began to drop. His skin was wet and clammy and his face was pale. He began to emanate an odor that can only be described as sickness. I don't recall when, but I ordered a room deodorizer. I am sure you can see that on my bill. When the nurses took his temperature, they said it was normal.

On Sunday morning, December 17th, I called Dr. S's office, and got his service. Later that day, his partner, Dr. R, called and visited at the hospital. He ordered up some x-rays of John's abdomen. He said these showed a small blockage, an obstruction in the small bowel. He said it was small, and shouldn't cause John as much distress as he was experiencing. He said my husband was overreacting, and he couldn't understand why. Dr. T cheerfully said an obstruction could be the cause of all John's symptoms. I stopped listening to Dr. T at that point. John was panting, his heart was racing, his blood pressure was dropping, his respiration was way up, his skin was clammy, his stomach was distended, he smelled, but they thought he was overreacting.

I don't doubt that Dr. S did everything right surgically. I believe that's probably the case. But medically there was not enough done to get my husband through this ordeal. I later learned that someone who is immuno-suppressed, as my husband would be, coming off of chemotherapy and radiation, wouldn't have elevated white blood cell counts to indicate infection. Could this be the reason that infection wasn't considered, that his white cells didn't rise? If so, that was a major oversight on their part. And of course, in retrospect, there were all those other symptoms of raging infection . . . but who was watching? Not Dr. S, who left John for the entire weekend in the care of this neophyte Dr. T, neither one of whom could deduce infection. Not the nurses, who were mostly devoting their time to planning their unit's Christmas party, or doing their Christmas shopping on-line on their computers at the nurse's station. Yes, I was watching and seething . . .

In any case, that is the focus of this suit, neglect and medical malpractice, even if the surgical component wasn't at fault.

Despite the fact that this woman proved to be a wonderful advocate for her husband, her pleas fell on deaf and insensitive ears. I have heard physicians, exasperated that their patients were failing, blame the patient for not sucking it up and taking the discomfort like a man. In reviewing the hospital records, it became abundantly clear that, after having the piece of colon removed, his intestines went to sleep and stopped working. This is common for most who have surgery and it occurs for just a few days after colon surgery. By the way, there was no residual cancer. While the doctors were writing in their notes that the patient was doing well, they probably never took note of the fact that this patient was taking large doses of narcotics, three and four times a day, for what he described was severe pain (8 to 10 on a pain scale of 10).

On the ninth day postoperatively he still had not passed gas and still could not drink any liquid. Had x-rays or a CT scan been done, and it should have been done for anyone suffering for more than just a few days, it would have revealed the intestinal obstruction that was causing the pain. On the tenth day, he developed a high fever. No cultures or evaluation of any kind were done. On the eleventh day postoperatively, his blood pressure dropped and he went into shock. The next morning, a CT scan was ordered and showed the obstruction. He was brought to the operating room and died on the table.

His surgeon and hospital staff will deny any fault. There will be a long and expensive court battle. And it is anyone's guess as to the outcome. The bottom line is that many mistakes were made, many signs of a problem were ignored, and it resulted in an unnecessary death. To the medical world—and the rest of the world—this patient is just one more statistic. And keeping things as statistics keeps us at arm's length from the heart of the problem. The fact is, a *man* died that day, not a statistic. He did not just expire. He was not a carton of milk. He was a husband, a father, a son, and an American citizen. And his life was taken from him by a system that is failing.

Over 90,000 people a year, dead from medical error (of course Health-Grades says 200,000). The equivalent of a jumbo jet full of people crashing and killing everyone on board—nearly every day of the year.

In the time it's taken you to read this chapter, three more patients have died from preventable medical malpractice.

How many more unnecessary mistakes, maimings, and deaths will it take before we say enough is enough? The power for change is in your hands now. And it starts by taking back control of your own health care, becoming a proactive participant in every aspect of it—from diet and lifestyle, to research and education, questioning everything until you get satisfactory answers, and establishing a medical plan of action for you and your loved ones *before* you need it. And while you are at it, you can call or write your representative in Congress too and demand that these public servants start serving the public instead of their own special interests.

There is one patient hanging on for dear life in intensive care—the medical system. But it is not too late to save it. We have wiped out smallpox, put a man on the moon, and helped to tear down the Berlin Wall. We can build the greatest health care system in the world. But we have to want it badly enough. Then we have to do whatever it takes to make it happen. You might be thinking, "Slow down, I'm just reading this book to make sure that *I* don't become a statistic!" And that's okay. Reading this book is a great start. And taking care of yourself and your loved ones is the most important thing you can do. Not only does it set a great example, but as we become a society of healthy, conscious, empowered citizens, there is no limit to what we can do together. There is plenty of evidence that sustained focus and public reporting, among other things, seem to make a significant difference in the quality of health care, especially in the area of patient safety. As HealthGrades stated: "Because of the positive effects of public reporting and the continued lack of a national cohesive and consistent structure to identify, analyze, report and share critical quality and patient safety information, it is imperative that the development and dissemination of highly visible consumer guides and public performance reporting be a priority for consumers."[13]

Please keep me informed on your progress. And be well. To Your Health!

NOTES

INTRODUCTION

1. Rosenfield, Harvey, *Silent Violence. Silent Death. A Consumer's Guide to the Medical Malpractice Epidemic*. Washington, DC: Essential Books, 1994.

2. Rosenfeld, *Silent Violence*.

3. Linda T. Kohn, Janet M. Corrigan, and Molla S. Donaldson, eds. *To Err Is Human: Building a Safe Health System* (Washington, DC: National Academy Press, 2000), 1.

4. Kohn, Corrigan, and Donaldson, *To Err Is Human*, 27.

5. Federal Aviation Association, www.faa.gov/data_research/accident_incident/ (retrieved May 24, 2009); www.faa.gov/search/?q=airline+passenger+accident+statistics (retrieved May 24, 2009).

6. American Hospital Association, "Fast Facts on US Hospitals," *AHA Resource Center* 2007, www.aha.org/aha/resource-center/Statistics-and-Studies/fast-facts.html (retrieved May 21, 2009).

7. Medical Practice, "National Medical Practice Statistics," ExpertHub Network 2009, www.medicalmalpractice.com/National-Medical-malpractice-Facts.cfm (retrieved March 3, 2009); R. A. Reynolds, J. A. Rizzo, and M. L. Gonzalez, "The Cost of Medical Professional Liability," *Journal of the American Medical Association* 257 (1987): 2776–81; "Doctors, Fearing Liability Suits, Resign," *Physician's Financial News* (1997): 47.

8. National Center for Health Statistics, www.cdc.gov/nchs/nvss.htm (retrieved May 21, 2009).

CHAPTER 1

1. www.quotegarden.com/medical.html (retrieved February 8, 2009).

2. Jason Lazarou, "Incidence of Adverse Drug Reactions in Hospitalized Patients," *Journal of American Medical Association* 229, no. 15 (April 1998): 1200; Thomas J. Moore, "Time to Act on Drug Safety," *Journal of the American Medical Associations* 279 (May 1998): 1571; Todd Zwillich, "Drug Errors Injure 1.5 Million Annually," WebMD, http://aolsvc.health.webmd.aol.com/content/Article/125/115943.htm?pagenumbers=2 (retrieved August 6, 2006); Reshma Kapadia, "Ten Things Your Hospital Won't Tell You," *Smart Money* (1996), www.smartmoney.com/spending/rip-offs/10-things-your-hospital-wont-tell-you-20059/ (retrieved January 7, 2008); David Bates, "Relationship between Medical Errors and Adverse Drug Reactions," *Journal of General Internal Medicine* 10, no. 4 (April 1995): 199–205; D. W. Bates et al., "Incidence of Adverse Drugs Events and Potential Adverse Drug Events: Implications for Prevention," *Journal of the American Medical Association* 274 (July 1995): 29–34.

CHAPTER 2

1. www.quotegarden.com/medical.html (retrieved February 8, 2009)

2. Soeren Mattke, et al., "Health Care Quality Indicators Project: Initial Indicators Report," March 2006, OECD Health Papers No. 22, World Health Organization and its Update (October 2006).

3. HealthGrades. "HealthGrades Quality Study: Patient Safety in American Hospitals," HealthGrades, July 2004, www.healthgrades.com/media/English/pdf/hg_patient_safety_Study_final.pdf (retrieved May 24, 2009). Out of 5,000 hospitals studied, only 250 were rated five star. That is approximately 5 percent of the nation's hospitals that provide excellent care. The report describes the poor outcomes in the one- and three-star hospitals.

4. H. Burstin, S. R. Lipsitz, and T. A. Brennan, "Socio-economic Status and Risk for Substandard Medical Care," *Journal of the American Medical Association* 268 (November 1992): 2387.

5. J. Barg, "HMO Medical Director Becomes Critic," *Physician's News Digest* (December 1998).

6. Fathie, "Healthcare for the Healthy," *American Academy of Neurological and Orthopedic Surgeons.* www.aanos.org/jnoms.htm (retrieved May 21, 2009).

7. The refusal of insuring individuals or not insuring preexisting conditions varies from state to state (there is no federal law). Insurance carriers in New York State have the right to refuse coverage of preexisting conditions if the individual has not had insurance coverage for sixty-three consecutive days. New York State insurance carriers may allow some individuals to pay extra for a rider to cover those preexisting conditions. Many states still have the right to refuse coverage: New York State Insurance Law #4318 (McKinney's *Consolidated Law of New York*, 2000). www.ins.state.ny.us/ogco2002/rg021116.htm (retrieved May 21, 2009).

8. Martin Gaynor, James B. Rebitzer, and Lowell J. Taylor. "Physician Incentives in Health Maintenance Organizations," *Journal of Political Economy* 112, no. 4 (August 2004): 915–31.

9. Linda Sage, "Managed Care Incentives Should Be Disclosed," *Bio-Medicine* 27 (January 1999), http://news.bio-medicine.org/medicine-news-2/Managed-Care-Incentives-Should-Be-Disclosed (retrieved April 29, 2009); www.sage@medicine.wustl.edu (retrieved May 18, 2009).

10. News-Medical.Net, "Cigna Reach Agreement on Physician Ranking System," October 30, 2007, www.news-medical.net/print_article.asp?id=31931 (retrieved April 25, 2009).

11. Author's personal communications with doctors working for HMOs.

12. Job description: Nexus Healthcare: www.nexushc.com.

13. Editorial, "Gouging Women on Health Insurance," *New York Times*, 3 November, 2008, p. A30, www.nytimes.com/2008/11/03/opinion/03mon2.html (retrieved May 21, 2009).

14. National Women's Law Center, "Nowhere to Turn," www.nwlc.org/archive.cfm?section=archive (retrieved April 8, 2009).

15. Medicare Services: www.CMShhs.gov/MLNProducts/35_PreventiveServices.asp#TopOfPage (retrieved April 24, 2009). This states that Medicare will pay for only one Initial Preventive Physical Examination (IPPE), as a welcome to Medicare and has to be performed during the first six months of enrollment in Medicare. No labs, electrocardiograms, x-rays, or bone density tests will be covered. Thereafter, no preventive annual physicals will be covered.

16. Social Justice Research, *American Association of Retired People* 1, no. 3 (September 1987): 361–75; Stephanie Saul, "In Sour Economy, Some Scale Back on Medications," *New York Times*, October 21, 2008; Tatiana Harrison, "Falling into the Gap: How Medicare Part D Fails People with Rheumatoid Arthritis," September 7, 2008, www.healthmad.com/Healthcare-Industry/Falling-Into-the-Gap-How-Medicare-Part-D-Fails-People-with-Rheumatoid-Arthritis.243601 (retrieved February 24, 2009); Terry Emerick, "Part D: Rx for Disaster," *ePluibusMedia* (May 12, 2006), www.epluribusmedia.org/archives/features/2006/0511part_d.html (retrieved December 16, 2008).

17. LoveToKnowCorp, www.lovetoknow.com (retrieved January 2, 2009).

CHAPTER 3

1. www.quotegarden.com/medical.html (retrieved February 8, 2009).

2. Deborah Maliver, "Hospital Infections—Negligent Prevention and Treatment," *Biancheria and Maliver, PC* (2009), www.bem-law.com/PracticeAreas/Negligent-Treatment-of-Infection.asp (retrieved May 21, 2009); James Newfield, "Current Issues in Providing Wound Care in the Home," *Home Health Care Management* 17, no. 3 (2005): 233–42.

3. L. L. Leape, T. A. Brennan, N. Laird, et al., "The Nature of Adverse Events in Hospital Patients," *New England Journal of Medicine* 324, no. 6 (February 1991): 377–84; Eric J. Thomas and Troyen A. Brennan, "Incidence and Types of Preventable Adverse Events in Elderly Patients: Population Based Review of Medical Records," *British Medicine Journal* 320 (March 2000): 741–44; A. Gawande, E. J. Thomas, M. J. Zinner, and T. A. Brennan,

"The Incidence and Nature of Surgical Adverse Events in Colorado and Utah in 1992," *Surgery* 126 (July 1999): 66–75.

4. "Medical Malpractice," Insurance Information Institute 2009, www.iii.org/media/hottopics/insurance/medicalmal (retrieved April 28, 2009); Gary McAbee, "Lessons Can Be Learned from Malpractice Cases Involving Meningitis," *American Academy of Pediatrics APP News* 24, no. 4 (April 2004): 180–82; Gary N. McAbee, Charles Deitschel, and Jan Berger, "Pediatric Medicolegal Education in the 21st Century," *Pediatrics* 117, no. 5 (May 2006): 1790–92.

5. Deanna L. Reising and Patricia N. Allen, "Protecting Yourself from Malpractice Claims," *American Nurse Today* 2, no. 2 (February 2007): 39–43.

6. Insurance Information Institute, Inc., "Medical Malpractice: The Topic."

7. Editorial, "When Doctors Hide Medical Errors," *New York Times*, September 9, 2006, www.nytimes.com2006/09/09/opinion/09sat4.html?_r=2&oref=slogin (retrieved January 23, 2009).

8. Editorial, *New York Times*, "When Doctors Hide."

9. My personal fact sheets for two malpractice companies. PRI and MLMC—Physicians' Reciprocal Insurers, *Claims-Made Professional Liability Coverage*. Manhasset, NY: PRI and MLMC—Physicians' Reciprocal Insurers, 1995. 6

10. Insurance Information Institute, Inc., "Medical Malpractice: The Topic."

11. Insurance Information Institute, Inc., "Medical Malpractice: The Topic."

12. Robert S. Lagasse, Ellen S. Steinberg, Robert I. Katz, and Albert J. Saubermann, "Defining Quality of Perioperative Care by Statistical Process Control of Adverse Outcomes," *Anesthesiology* 82, no. 5 (May 1995): 1181–88; Gregory A. Nuttall, Linda Stehling, Christopher Beighley, and Ronald J. Faust, "Current Transfusion Practices of Members of the American Society of Anesthesiologists: A Survey," *Anesthesiology* 99, no. 6 (December 2003): 1433–43.

13. "Medical Malpractice Lawsuits Not the Cause of Health Care Crisis," *Public Citizen* 2007, www.citizen.org/pressroom/release.cfm?ID=2351 (retrieved March 19, 2009); Seth Oldmixon, *Public Citizen Congress Watch 2007,* Washington, DC: Public Citizen's Congress Watch, 2007; Charles Kuffner, "Bad Doctors Cause Lawsuits . . . Who Knew," Offthekuff.com 2005, www.offthekuff.com/mt/archives/004719.html (retrieved December 17, 2008).

14. Reising and Allen, "Protecting Yourself."

15. M. Williams, et al., "Inadequate Functional Literacy Among Patients at Two Public Health Hospitals," *Journal of the American Medical Association* 274, no. 21 (1995): 1677–82; Edward Rabinowitz, "Low Health Literacy Hits Physicians Where It Hurts," *Physician's Money Digest*, June 4, 2008.

16. *USA Today*, "Study: Off Label Drugs Often Prescribed," *USA Today*, May 8, 2006.

CHAPTER 4

1. www.quotegarden.com/medical.html (retrieved February 8, 2009).

2. Centers for Disease Control, www.cdc.gov/nchs/births (retrieved May 2, 2009).

3. Shelley Hitz, "Obesity in America: The Growing Epidemic," www.ambafrance-do.org/weight-loss/5961.php (retrieved May 24, 2009).

4. Elisa Elizabeth King Terry, "Do Increasing Rates of Autism in California Let Vaccines Off the Hook?," *Associated Content,* January 9, 2008, www.associatedcontent.com/article/531079/do_increasing_rates_of_autism_in_california.html?cat=70 (retrieved May 24, 2009).

CHAPTER 5

1. www.quotegarden.com/medical.html (retrieved February 8, 2009).

2. Zwillich, "Drug Errors."

3. Health and Science, "Cause of Deaths: Sloppy Doctors." *Time,* January 15, 2007, http://www.time.com/time/health/article/0,8599,1578074,00.html

4. Health and Science, *Time.*

5. "Comparison of Methods for Detecting Medication Errors in 36 Hospitals and Skilled Nursing Facilities." *American Journal of Health Systems: Pharmacy,* 50 (5): 436–46.

6. Zwillich, "Drug Errors."

7. Health and Science, *Time.*

8. Zwillich, "Drug Errors."

9. CRS News, "US: Pharmaceutical Industry Guidelines for Research Disclosure," *Business Respect,* 76 (July 9, 2004), www.businessrespect.net/page.php?Story_ID=1302 (retrieved May 24, 2009).

10. Florida law, section 456.42 Florida statutes, www.citizen.org/documents/FL_NPDB. pdf (retrieved May 18, 2009).

CHAPTER 6

1. Robert W. Derlet and John R. Richards, "Overcrowding in the Nation's Emergency Departments: Complex Causes and Disturbing Effects," *Annals of Emergency Medicine* 35 (January 2000): 63–68.

2. Richard J. Ackerman, Kathy A. Kemle, Robert L. Vogle, and Ralph C. Griffin, "Emergency Department Use by Nursing Homes," *Annals of Emergency Medicine* 31 (June 1998): 749–57.

3. Joel Cohen, *ER: Enter at Your Own Risk,* Far Hills, NJ: New Horizon Press, 2001.

4. Cohen, *ER: Enter at Your Own Risk.*

5. Robert Reinhold, "Crisis in Emergency Rooms: More Symptoms than Cures," *New York Times,* July 28, 1988, p. 1A.

6. Institutes of Medicine. "Report on Emergency Medical Services." *Institute of Medicine* 2006. www.iom. edu/?id=48898 (retrieved May 21, 2009).

7. R. H. Mehta and K. A. Eagle, "Missed Diagnosis of Acute Coronary Syndromes in the Emergency Room: Continuing Challenges," *New England Journal of Medicine* 342 (April 2000): 1207–10.

8. Mehta and Eagle, "Missed Diagnosis."

9. Cohen, *ER: Enter at Your Own Risk.*

10. Cohen, *ER: Enter at Your Own Risk.*

11. Institute of Medicine, "Report on Emergency Medical Services."

12. Cohen, *ER: Enter at Your Own Risk.*

13. Dennis Alfaro, M. Andrew Levitt, David English, Virgil Williams, and Ronald Eisenberg, "Accuracy of Interpretation of CT Scans in an Emergency Medicine Residency Program," *Annals of Emergency Medicine* 25, no. 2 (February 1995): 169–74.

14. Cohen, *ER: Enter at Your Own Risk.*

15. Institute of Medicine, "Report on Emergency Medical Services."

16. Cohen, *ER: Enter at Your Own Risk.*

17. Leape, et al., "The Nature of Adverse Events."

18. Mayo Clinic Staff, "Stroke: Definition." Mayo Clinic, July 3, 2008, www.mayoclinic.com/health/stroke/DS00150 (retrieved May 24, 2009); Mayo Clinic Staff, "Stroke: Treatment," Mayo Clinic, July 3, 2008, www.mayoclinic.com/health/stroke-treatment/BN00056 (retrieved May 24, 2009).

19. Cohen, *ER: Enter at Your Own Risk.*

CHAPTER 7

1. Bureau of Vital Statistics. cdc.gov/nchs/fastats/deaths/htm.

2. Salvador Borges-Neto, "Assessing Patients with Nuclear Imaging," June 19, 2002. Updated March 24, 2003, http://cme.medscape.com/viewarticle/436816 (retrieved April 27, 2009).

3. Sripal Bangalore, Siu-Sun Yao, and Farooq A. Chaudhry, "Role of Left Atrial Size in Risk Stratification and Prognosis of Patients Undergoing Stress Echocardiography," *Journal of the American College of Cardiology* 50 (June 2007): 1254–62.

4. Antonio Colombo, "Drug Releasing Stents Showing Higher Complication Rates," *Bio-Medicine* 2003, http://news.bio-medicine.org/medicine-news-3/Drug-releasing-stents-showing-higher-complication-rate-than-clinical-trials-indicated-10129-1/ (retrieved May 23, 2009).

5. Colombo, "Drug Releasing Stents."

6. Roni Caryn Rabin, "Heart Stents Found as Effective as Bypass for Many Patients," *New York Times,* February 20, 2009.

7. Gerald Fletcher, Gary J. Balady, Ezra A. Amsterdam, et al., "Exercise Standards for Testing and Training: A Statement for Healthcare Professionals From the American Heart Association, *Circulation* 104 (2001): 1694.

8. E. Lonn, S. Yusuf, M. J. O. Arnold, et al., "Homocysteine Lowering with Folic Acid and B Vitamins in Vascular Disease: The Heart Outcomes Prevention Evaluation (HOPE) 2 Investigators," *New England Journal of Medicine* 354, no. 15. (April 13, 2006): 1567–77.

9. Lancet, "Effect of Ramipril on Mortality and Morbidity of Survivors of Acute Myocardial Infarction with Clinical Evidence of Heart Failure. The Acute Infarction Ramipril Efficacy (AIRE) Study Investigators," *Lancet* 342, no. 8875 (October 2, 1993): 821–28.

10. Lonn, et al., "Homocysteine Lowering with Folic Acid."

11. Lonn, et al., "Homocysteine Lowering with Folic Acid."

CHAPTER 8

1. Joint Commission of Hospitals, www.jointcommission.org.

2. National Cancer Center, http://ganjoho.ncc.go.jp/pro/statistics/en/graph_db_index.html (March 24, 2009).

3. glgroup.com/news/overview_of_the_nutritional_supplements_market_10/82.html.

CHAPTER 9

1. Duke Health, www.dukehealth/devil.studentaffairs.duke.edu/health_info/pelvin%20examination.html. (retrieved May 24, 2009).

2. Silverman & Fodera, Pap smear litigation, www.civilrights.com/PapSmearLitigation.php (retrieved May 23, 2009); www.civilrights.com/CancerinWomen.php (retrieved May 24, 2009).

3. Amy Scholten, "Human Papillomavirus Testing," Beth Israel Deaconess Medical Center, www.bidmc.org/YourHealth/MedicalProcedures.aspx?ChunkID=32308 (retrieved May 23, 2009).

4. Mayo Clinic Staff, "Cervical Cancer: Tests and Diagnosis," Mayo Clinic June 29, 2007, www.mayoclinic.com/health/cervical-cancer/DS00167/DSECTION=tests-and-diagnosis (retrieved May 21, 2009).

5. Gordon Gibb, "The Gardasil Vaccine Issue: The Tail that Wags the Dog?" Lawyers and Settlements, August 21, 2008, www.lawyersandsettlements.com/features/gardasil-gardisal-vaccine.html (retrieved May 21, 2009).

6. U.S. Cancer Statistics Working Group, "United States Cancer Statistics: 1999–2005 Incidence and Mortality Web-based Report," Atlanta: Department of Health and Human Services, Centers for Disease Control and Prevention, and National Cancer Institute, 2009, www.cdc.gov/uscs (retrieved May 24, 2009). Cervical Cancer Statistics, www.cdc.gov/cancer/cervical/statistics/ (retrieved May 23, 2009).

7. Cervical Cancer Statistics.

8. National Institutes of Health, "Consensus Development Conference Statement: Cervical Cancer," NIH Consensus Statement Online 1996 April 1–3, 43, no. 1 (1996): 1–38. http://consensus.nih.gov/1996/1996CervicalCancer102html.htm (retrieved May 24, 2009).

9. "Benefits of HPV Vaccine Questioned, Los Angeles Times, July 15, 2008; Charlotte Haug, "Human Papillomavirus Vaccination—Reasons for Caution," New England Journal of Medicine 359, no. 8 (August 21, 2008): 861–62.

10. Aruna D. Pradhan, JoAnn E. Manson, Jacques E. Rossouw, et al., "Inflammatory Biomarkers, Hormone Replacement Therapy, and Incident Coronary Heart Disease: Prospective Analysis from the Women's Health Initiative Observational Study," Journal of the American Medical Association 288, no. 8 (August 2002): 980–87; Susan M. Gapstur, Monica Morrow, and Thomas A. Sellers, "Hormone Replacement Therapy and Risk of Breast Cancer With a Favorable Histology: Results of the Iowa Women's Health Study," Journal of the American Medical Association 281, no. 22 (June 9, 1999): 2091–97.

11. American College of Obstetrics and Gynecology and the American Academy of Pediatrics, January 31, 2003, www.acog.org/from_home/publications/press_releases/nr01-31-1.

12. American College of Obstetrics and Gynecology, November 3, 2006, micra_org/womens_health/docs/acog_news_news_release_womens_atc.pdf.

CHAPTER 10

1. www.quotegarden.com/medical.html (retrieved February 8, 2009).

2. Mayo Clinic Staff, "Trichinosis: Causes," Mayo Clinic, February 1, 2008, www.mayoclinic.com/health/trichinosis/DS00689/DSECTION=causes (retrieved May 21, 2009).

CHAPTER 11

1. Wikipedia, "Doctor of Medicine," http://en.wikipedia.org/wiki/M.D. (retrieved May 21, 2009).

2. Joseph Biederman, Michael C. Monuteaux, Thomas Spencer, et al., "Stimulant Therapy and Risk for Subsequent Substance Use Disorders in Male Adults With ADHD: A Naturalistic Controlled 10-Year Follow-Up Study," *American Journal of Psychiatry* 165, no. 5 (May 2008): 597–603.

3. A. Poulton, "Growth on Stimulant Medication: Clarifying the Confusion: A Review." *Archive of Disease in Childhood* 90, no. 8 (August 2005): 801–6.

4. Michael Grunebaum, Steven Ellis, Shuhua Li, Maria Oquendo, and J. John Mann, "Anti-Depressants and Suicide Risk in the United States, 1985–1999," *Journal of Clinical Psychiatry* 65, no. 11 (November 2004): 1456–62. http://excalibur.cpmc.columbia.edu/reprints/Grunebaum%20et%20al%20JCP%202003.pdf (retrieved May 22, 2009).

5. Benjamen Grasso, "Errors in Psychiatry," *Medscape Psychiatry and Mental Health*, June 29, 2007.

CHAPTER 12

1. www.quotegarden.com/medical.html (retrieved February 8, 2009).

CHAPTER 13

1. www.quotegarden.com/medical.html (retrieved February 8, 2009).

2. Kohn, Corrigan, and Donaldson, *To Err Is Human*.

3. Public Citizen Press Room, "Kentucky Doctors Not Facing a Medical Malpractice Insurance Crisis, Public Citizen Report Shows: Biggest Health Problem

Is the 4.7 Percent of Kentucky Doctors Who Are Responsible for 50 Percent of Medical Malpractice Payouts to Injured Patients," February 4, 2004, http://www .citizen.org/pressroom/Release.cfm.ID=1640 (retrieved May 18, 2009).

4. Kohn, Corrigan, and Donaldson, *To Err Is Human.*

5. Public Citizen Press Room.

6. Harvey Rosenfeld, *Silent Violence, Silent Death: A Consumer's Guide to the Medical Malpractice Epidemic*, Washington, DC: Essential Books, 1994.

7. Rosenfeld, *Silent Violence, Silent Death.*

8. HealthGrades, *HealthGrade Quality Study*, July 2004.

9. For their latest reports on your hospital or physician, go to www.healthgrades.com.

10. Richard P. Wenzel and Michael B. Edmond, "The Impact of Hospital Acquired Blood Stream Infection," *Center for Disease Control Special Issue* 7, no. 2 (March–April 2001).

11. Michael J. Berens, "Infectious Epidemic Carves Deadly Path: Poor Hygiene, Overwhelmed Workers Contribute to Thousands of Deaths," *Chicago Tribune*, July 21, 2002.

12. Michael J. Berens, "Hospitals' Hidden Killers: More Germs Are Taking Patients Lives," *Seattle Times*, July 25, 2002.

13. "Medicine's Dirty Little Secret: Hospitals Promote Doctors to Wash Their Hands," *Washington Post*, September 30, 1997.

14. Jessica Pasley, "Nursing Shortage Hurts Patients," *Reporter: Vanderbilt Medical Center's Weekly Newspaper,* April 27, 2001, www.mc.vanderbilt.edu/reporter/index. html?ID=1480 (retrieved May 24, 2009).

15. HealthGrades, "The Eleventh Annual HealthGrades Hospital Quality in America Study," October 2008 HealthGrades, "The Seventh Annual HealthGrades Hospital Quality and Clinical Excellence Study," January 2009, http://healthgrades com/media/DMS/pdf/ HospitalQualityClinicalExcellenceStudy2009.pdf (retrieved May 24, 2009).

16. HealthGrades, "HealthGrades Quality Study: Fourth Annual Patient Safety in American Hospitals Study," April 2007, http://healthgrades.com/media/DMS/pdf/PatientSafetyIn AmericanHospitalsStudy2007.pdf (retrieved May 24, 2009).

17. For example, www.hospitalcompare.hhs.gov.

CHAPTER 14

1. www.quotegarden.com/medical.html (retrieved February 8, 2009).

2. Paul Ian Tartter, David Pace, Mark Frost, and Jonine L. Bernstein, "Delay in Diagnosis of Breast Cancer," *Annals of Surgery* 229, no. 1 (January 1999): 91–96.

3. Pamela F. Gallin and Joseph K. Vetter. "Gambling with Your Life," *Readers Digest* (August 2006).

4. Gallin and Vetter, "Gambling with Your Life."

5. Gallin and Vetter, "Gambling with Your Life."

6. Gallin and Vetter, "Gambling with Your Life."

CHAPTER 15

1. www.quotegarden.com/medical.html (retrieved February 8, 2009).

2. L. McFarland and P. Bernasconi, "*Saccharomyces boulardii*: A Review of an Innovative Biotherapeutic Agent," *Microbial Ecology in Health and Disease* 6, no. 4 (July 1993): 157–71.

3. G. Centini-Sauri and G. Sierra Basto, "Therapeutic Evaluation of *Saccharomyces boulardii* in Children with Acute Diarrhea," *Annals of Pediatrics* 41 (1994): 397–400.

CHAPTER 16

1. www.quotelucy.com/quotes/senator-john-kerry-quotes-6.html (retrieved May 24, 2009).

2. Lea Winerman, "The Uninsured in America," *Online NewsHour*, April 6, 2007, www.pbs.org/newshour/indepth_coverage/health/uninsured/whoaretheuninsured.html (retrieved May 24, 2009).

3. Karen Davis, "President's Message: 2003 Annual Report: Achieving a High Performance Health System," Commonwealth Fund, www.commonwealthfund.org/annreprt/2003/pdf/Report_01_msg_pres.pdf (retrieved May 22, 2009).

4. Julie Appleby, "Child Health Care Varies Widely among States, Report Shows," *USA Today* (May 28, 2008): 5B.

5. American Medical Student Association, "Theoretical Models for Delivering Healthcare," www.amsa.org/uhc/theories.cfm (retrieved May 24, 2009); www.amsa.org/business (retrieved May 24, 2009).

6. Voice for the Uninsured, "The Health Care Crisis: Overview of the American Medical Association: Reform Proposal," 2008, www.voicefortheuninsured.org/pdf/proposal overview.pdf (retrieved January 28, 2009).

7. Dennis Kucinich, "Universal Health Care," Kucinich for President 2008, http://kucinich.us/issues/universalhealth.php (retrieved June 28, 2007).

8. Philip Musgrove, Riadh Zeramdini, and Guy Carrin, "Basic Patterns in National Health Expenditures," *Bulletin of the World Health Organization* 80, no. 2 (February 2002): 134–42.

9. Kucinich, "Universal Health Care."

10. Hillary Clinton and Barack Obama, "Making Patient Safety the Centerpiece of Medical Liability Reform," *New England Journal of Medicine* 354 (May 2006): 2205–8.

11. Lynn Langton and Thomas Cohen, "Civil Bench and Jury Trials in State Court, 2005," U.S. Department of Justice: Office of Justice Programs: 2005, www.ojp.usdoj.gov/bjs/pub/pdf/cbjtsc05.pdf (retrieved May 23, 2009).

12. David M. Studdert, Michelle M. Mello, Atul A. Gawande, et al., "Claims, Errors, and Compensation Payments in Medical Malpractice Litigation," *New England Journal of Medicine* 354, no. 19 (May 2006): 2024–33.

13. HealthGrades, Health Grades Quality Study, July 2004.

RESOURCES

GENERAL MEDICAL INFORMATION

- National Library of Medicine (the largest medical library in the world) will supply articles on any topic: www.custserv@nlm.nih.gov
- The same library has links to many other services: www.nlm.nih.gov
- For information on any condition or medical topic, go to: www.drkoop.com/conditions/ency
- For up-to-date information on diseases: www.cdc.gov
- Timely reviews of health topics: www.healthline.com
- The Agency for Healthcare Research and Quality supplies information on health care quality, cost, errors, and outcomes: www.ahcpr.gov/qual/errorsix.htm
- The American Medical Association provides updated medical information: www.ama-assn.org/ama/pub/category3457.html
- MEDEM's Medical Library: www.medem.com/medlb/medlb_entry.cfm
- The American Academy of Pediatrics offers up-to-date information: www.aap.org
- For prevention of medication errors in hospitalized children, go to: www.aap.org/policy/re9751.html
- The Institutes of Medicine provides health and science policies: www.iom.edu
- The Society of Health System Pharmacists' document "Preventing Medication errors in Hospitals": www.ashp.com/bestpractices/medmis/guide/preventing.pdf

- The American Board of Medical Specialists lists all board certified members: www.abms.org
- For help in choosing a physician or hospital: www.castleconnolley.com
- For legal help: www.nolo.com

HOSPITAL INFORMATION

- HealthGrades gives up-to-date information, rating all hospitals in the United States: healthgrades.com
- American Hospital Association: www.hospitalconnect.com/aha/resource_center/index.html
- The National Center for Health Statistics: www.nchsquery2cdc.gov
- The National Institute of Mental Health: www.nimh.info@nih.gov
- The American Medical Association offers hospital and doctor finders: www.ama-assn.org
- The following Web page helps patients find the best doctors and hospitals: www.bestdoctors.com

INFORMATION ON INSURANCE

- Health Allies helps individuals find affordable health care services, whether they have insurance or not: www.healthallies.com
- The American Association of Retired Persons offers information, especially for those over 50 years of age: www.aarp.org

FOR CANCER-RELATED ISSUES

- Contact the National Cancer Institute: www.cancercenters.cancer.gov
- The American College of Surgeons has a dedicated Web site for cancer issues: www.facs.org/cancerprogram/howto.html
- The National Cancer Institute is part of the government's Web site: www.cancer.gov
- The American Cancer Society site: www.cancer.com

FOR STROKE VICTIMS OR HEART-RELATED ISSUES

- www.americanheart.org/statistics
- www.stroke.org

- www.stokecenter.org
- The National Heart, Lung and Blood Institute offers up-to-date information: www.nhlbi.nih.gov

Finally, there are three Web sites that explain why and how tests are done, as well as the explanation of surgical procedures, in easy to understand language:

- www.adam.com
- www.yoursurgery.com
- www.health.discovery.com/diseaseandcond/encyclopediamedical_tests_encclopedia.html

BIBLIOGRAPHY

Ackerman, Richard J., Kathy A. Kemle, Robert L. Vogle, and Ralph C. Griffin. "Emergency Department Use by Nursing Homes." *Annals of Emergency Medicine* 31 (June 1998): 749–57.

Alfaro, Dennis, M., Andrew Levitt, David English, Virgil Williams, and Ronald Eisenberg. "Accuracy of Interpretation of CT Scans in an Emergency Medicine Residency Program." *Annals of Emergency Medicine* 25, no. 2 (February 1995): 169–74.

American Association of Retired People. "Social Justice Research." *American Association of Retired People* 1, no. 3 (September 1987): 361–75.

American Hospital Association. "Fast Facts on US Hospitals." AHA Resource Center 2007. www.aha.org/aha/resource-center/Statistics-and-Studies/fast-facts.html (retrieved May21, 2009).

American Medical Student Association. "Theoretical Models for Delivering Healthcare." www.amsa.org/uhc/theories.cfm; www.amsa.org/business (retrieved May 24, 2009).

Anderson, Gerard F., Uwe E. Reinhardt, Peter S. Hussey, and Varduhi Petrosyan. "It's the Prices, Stupid: Why the United States Is So Different from Other Countries." *Health Affairs* 22, no. 3 (May–June 2003): 89–105.

Appleby, Julie. "Child Health Care Varies Widely Among States, Report Shows." *USA Today* (May 28, 2008): 5B.

Bangalore, Sripal, Siu-Sun Yao, and Farooq A. Chaudhry. "Role of Left Atrial Size in Risk Stratification and Prognosis of Patients Undergoing Stress Echocardiography." *Journal of the American College of Cardiology* 50 (June 2007).

Barg, J. "HMO Medical Director Becomes Critic." *Physician's News Digest* (December 1998).

Bates, David. "Relationship between Medical Errors and Adverse Drug Reactions." *Journal of General Internal Medicine* 10, no. 4 (April 1995): 199–205.

Bates, D. W., D. J. Cullen, N. Laird, et al. "Incidence of Adverse Drugs Events and Potential Adverse Drug Events: Implications for Prevention." *Journal of the American Medical Association* 274 (July 1995): 29–34.

Berens, Michael J. "Hospitals' Hidden Killers: More Germs Are Taking Patients Lives." *Seattle Times,* July 25, 2002.

Berens, Michael J. "Infectious Epidemic Carves Deadly Path: Poor Hygiene, Overwhelmed Workers Contribute to Thousands of Deaths." *Chicago Tribune,* July 21, 2002.

Biederman, Joseph, Michael C. Monuteaux, Thomas Spencer, Timothy E. Wilens, Heather A. MacPherson, and Stephen V. Faraone. "Stimulant Therapy and Risk for Subsequent Substance Use Disorders in Male Adults with ADHD: A Naturalistic Controlled 10-Year Follow-Up Study." *American Journal of Psychiatry* 165, no. 5 (May 2008): 597–603.

Borges-Neto, Salvador. "Assessing Patients with Nuclear Imaging," June 19, 2002, updated March 24, 2003; http://cme.medscape.com/viewarticle/436816 (retrieved April 27, 2009).

Brilman, Judith, David Doezema, Dan Tandberg, David P. Sklar, Kathleen D. Davis, Shelby Simms, and Betty J. Skipper. "Triage: Limitations in Predicting Need for Emergent Care and Hospital Admission." *Annals of Emergency Medicine* 27, no. 3 (April 1996): 493–99.

Burstin, H., S. R. Lipsitz, and T. A. Brennan. "Socioeconomic Status and Risk for Substandard Medical Care." *Journal of the American Medical Association* 268 (November 1992): 2387.

CRS News. "US: Pharmaceutical Industry Guidelines for Research Disclosure," *Business Respect* 76 (July 9, 2004). www.businessrespect.net/page.php?Story_ID=1302 (retrieved May 24, 2009).

Centers for Disease Control. www.cdc.gov/nchs/births (retrieved May 2, 2009).

Centini-Sauri, G., and G. Sierra Basto. "Therapeutic Evaluation of *Saccharomyces boulardii* in Children with Acute Diarrhea." *Annals of Pediatrics* 41 (1994): 397–400.

Citizen.org. "Medical Malpractice Lawsuits Not the Cause of Health Care Crisis." Public Citizen 2007, www.citizen.org/pressroom/release.cfm?ID=2351 (retrieved March 19, 2009).

Clinton, Hillary, and Barack Obama. "Making Patient Safety the Centerpiece of Medical Liability Reform." *New England Journal of Medicine* 354 (May 2006): 2205–8.

Cohen, Joel. *ER: Enter at Your Own Risk.* Far Hills, NJ: New Horizon Press, 2001.

Colombo, Antonio. "Drug Releasing Stents Showing Higher Complication Rates." Bio-Medicine 2003. http://news.bio-medicine.org/medicine-news-3/Drug-releasing-stents-showing-higher-complication-rate-than-clinical-trials-indicated-10129-1/ (retrieved May 23, 2009).

Colorado Springs Gazette, September 16, 2002. "Comparison Methods for Detecting Errors" (retrieved May 21, 2009).

Davis, Karen. "President's Message: 2003 Annual Report: Achieving a High Performance Health System." Commonwealth Fund, 2003. www.Commonwealthfund.org/annreprt/2003/pdf/Report_01_msg_pres.pdf (retrieved May 22, 2009).

Derlet, Robert W., and John R. Richards. "Overcrowding in the Nation's Emergency Departments: Complex Causes and Disturbing Effects." *Annals of Emergency Medicine* 35 (January 2000): 63–68.

"Doctors, Fearing Liability Suits, Resign." *Physicians Financial News* (1992): 42.

Editorial. "Gouging Women on Health Insurance." *New York Times*, November 3, 2008, p. A30. www.nytimes.com/2008/11/03/opinion/03mon2.html (retrieved May 21, 2009).

Editorial. "When Doctors Hide Medical Errors." *New York Times*, September 9, 2006. www.nytimes.com2006/09/09/opinion/09sat4.html?_r=2&oref=slogin (retrieved January 23, 2009).

Emerick, Terry. "Part D: Rx for Disaster." ePluibusMedia, May 12, 2006. www.epluribus media.org/archives/features/2006/0511part_d.html (retrieved December 16, 2008).

Fathie. "Healthcare for the Healthy," American Academy of Neurological and Orthopedic Surgeons. www.aanos.org/jnoms.htm (retrieved May 21, 2009).

Federal Aviation Association. Accident incident report. www.faa.gov/data_research/ accident_incident/ (retrieved May 24, 2009).

Federal Aviation Association. Passenger accident statistics. www.faa.gov/search/ ?Q+airline+passeneger+accident+Statistics (retrieved May 24, 2009).

Fletcher, Gerald, Gary J. Balady, Ezra A. Amsterdam, Bernard Chaitman, Robert Eckel, Jerome Fleg, Victor F. Froelicher, Arthur S. Leon, et al. "Exercise Standards for Testing and Training: A Statement for Healthcare Professionals From the American Heart Association." *Circulation* 104 (2001): 1694

Folli, Hugo L., Robert L. Poole, William E. Benitz, and Juanita C. Russo. "Medication Error Prevention by Clinical Pharmacists in Two Children's Hospitals." *Pediatrics* 79, no. 5 (1987): 718–22.

Gallin, Pamela F., and Joseph K. Vetter. "Gambling with Your Life." *Readers Digest* (August 2006).

Gapstur, Susan M., Monica Morrow, and Thomas A. Sellers. "Hormone Replacement Therapy and Risk of Breast Cancer with a Favorable Histology: Results of the Iowa Women's Health Study." *Journal of the American Medical Association* 281, no. 22 (June 9, 1999): 2091–97.

Gawande, A., E. J. Thomas, M. J. Zinner, and T. A. Brennan. "The Incidence and Nature of Adverse Events in Colorado and Utah in 1992." *Surgery* 126 (July 1999): 66–75.

Gaynor, Martin, James B. Rebitzer, and Lowell J. Taylor. "Physician Incentives in Health Maintenance Organizations." *Journal of Political Economy* 112, no. 4 (August 2004): 915–31.

Gibb, Gordon. "The Gardasil Vaccine Issue: The Tail that Wags the Dog?" Lawyers and Settlements, August 21, 2008, www.lawyersandsettlements.com/features/gardasil-gardisal-vaccine.html (retrieved May 21, 2009).

Glaeser, Peter W., Jeff Linzer, Michael G. Tunik, Deborah Parkman Henderson, Jane Ball. "Survey of Nationally Registered Emergency Medical Services Providers: Pediatric Education." *Annals of Emergency Medicine* 36, no. 1 (July 2000): 33–38.

Grunebaum, Michael, Steven Ellis, Shuhua Li, Maria Oquendo, and J. John Mann. "Anti-Depressants and Suicide Risk in the United States, 1985–1999." *Journal of Clinical Psychiatry* 65, no. 11 (November 2004): 1456–62. http://excalibur.cpmc .columbia.edu/reprints/Grunebaum%20et%20al%20JCP%202003.pdf (retrieved May 22, 2009).

Haug, Charlotte. "Human Papillomavirus Vaccination—Reasons for Caution." *New England Journal of Medicine* 359, no. 8 (August 21, 2008): 861–62.

Harrison, Tatiana. "Falling into the Gap: How Medicare Part D Fails People with Rheumatoid Arthritis." Healthmad, September 7, 2008. www.healthmad.com/Healthcare-Industry/Falling-Into-the-Gap-How-Medicare-Part-D-Fails-People-with-Rheumatoid-Arthritis.243601 (retrieved February 24, 2009).

Health and Science. *Time*. January 15, 2007. [**AU**]http://search.time.com/results.html?N=0&Nty=1&Ntt=january+15%2C+2007 (retrieved May 24, 2009).

HealthGrades. "HealthGrades Quality Study: Fourth Annual Patient Safety in American Hospitals Study." April 2007. http://healthgrades.com/media/DMS/pdf /PatientSafetyInAmericanHospitalsStudy2007.pdf (retrieved May 24, 2009).

HealthGrades. "HealthGrades Quality Study: Patient Safety in American Hospitals." July 2004. http://healthgrades.com/media/english/pdf/hg_patient_safety_study_final.pdf (retrieved May 24, 2009).

HealthGrades. "The Eleventh Annual HealthGrades Hospital Quality In America Study." October 2008.

HealthGrades. "The Seventh Annual HealthGrades Hospital Quality and Clinical Excellence Study." January 2009. http://healthgrades.com/media/DMS/pdf/HospitalQualityClinicalExcellenceStudy2009.pdf (retrieved May 24, 2009).

Hitz, Shelley. "Obesity in America: The Growing Epidemic." www.ambafrancedo.org/weight-loss/5961.php (retrieved May 24, 2009).

Institute of Medicine. "Report on Emergency Medical Services." *Institute of Medicine* 2006 www.iom. edu/?id=48898 (retrieved May 21, 2009).

Insurance Information Institute. "Medical Malpractice: The Topic." January2009. www.iii.or/media/hottopics/insurance/medicalmal (retrieved April 28, 2009).

Kapadia, Reshma. "Ten Things Your Hospital Won't Tell You." Smart Money, 1996. www.smartmoney.com/spending/rip-offs/10-things-your-hospital-wont-tell-you-20059 (retrieved January 7, 2008).

Kelley, Ed. "Health, Spending and the Effort to Improve Quality in OECD Countries: A Review of the Data." *Journal of the Royal Society for the Promotion of Health* 127, no. 2 (March 2007): 64–71.

Kohn, Linda T., Janet M. Corrigan, and Molla S. Donaldson, eds. *To Err Is Human: Building a Safer Health System*. Washington, DC: National Academy Press, 2000.

Kucinich, Dennis. "Universal Health Care." Kucinich for President, 2008. www.kucinich.us/issues/universalhealth.php (retrieved June 28, 2007).

Kuffner, Charles. "Bad Doctors Cause Lawsuits . . . Who Knew." Offthekuff.com 2005, www.offthekuff.com/mt/archives/004719.html (retrieved December 17, 2008).

Lagasse, Robert S., Ellen S. Steinberg, Robert I. Katz, and Albert J. Saubermann. "Defining Quality of Perioperative Care by Statistical Process Control of Adverse Outcomes." *Anesthesiology* 82, no. 5 (May 1995): 1181–88.

Lancet. "Effect of Ramipril on Mortality and Morbidity of Survivors of Acute Myocardial Infarction with Clinical Evidence of Heart Failure. The Acute Infarction Ramipril Efficacy (AIRE) Study Investigators." *Lancet* 342, no. 8875 (October 2, 1993): 821–28.

Langton, Lynn, and Thomas Cohen. "Civil Bench and Jury Trials in State Court, 2005." U.S. Department of Justice: Office of Justice Programs, 2005. www.ojp.usdoj.gov/bjs/pub/pdf/cbjtsc05.pdf (retrieved May 23, 2009).

Lazarou, Jason. "Incidence of Adverse Drug Reactions in Hospitalized Patients." *Journal of the American Medical Association* 229, no. 15 (April 1998): 1200.

Leape, L. L., T. A. Brennan, N. Laird, A. G. Lawthers, A. R. Localio, B. A. Barnes, L. Hebert, J. P. Newhouse, P. C. Weiler, and H. Hiatt. "The Nature of Adverse Events in Hospital Patients." *New England Journal of Medicine* 324, no. 6 (February 1991): 377–84.

Lonn, E., S. Yusuf, M. J. O. Arnold, P. Sheridan, M. J. McQueen, J. Pogue, J. Probstfield, G. Fodor, C. Held, M. Micks, and J. Genest, Jr. "Homocysteine Lowering with Folic Acid and B Vitamins in Vascular Disease: The Heart Outcomes Prevention Evaluation (HOPE) 2 Investigators." *New England Journal of Medicine* 354, no. 15 (April 13, 2006): 1567–77.

LoveToKnowCorp. (2006-2009). www.lovetoknow.com (retrieved January 2, 2009).

Maliver, Deborah. "Hospital Infections—Negligent Prevention and Treatment." *Biancheria and Maliver, PC* 2009. www.bem-law.com/PracticeAreas/Negligent-Treatment-of-Infection.asp (retrieved May 21, 2009).

Mattke, Sorren, et al. "Health Care Quality Indicators Project: Initial Indicator Report." March 2006. OECD Health Working Paper No. 22, World Health Organization and its Update, October 2006.

Mayo Clinic Staff. July 25, 2007. www.mayoclinic.com/health/ (retrieved May 21, 2009).

Mayo Clinic Staff. "Cervical Cancer: Tests and Diagnosis." June 29, 2007. www.mayoclinic.com/health/cervical-cancer/DS00167/DSECTION=tests-and-diagnosis (retrieved May 21, 2009).

Mayo Clinic Staff. "Stroke: Definition." July 3, 2008. www.mayoclinic.com/health/stroke/DS00150 (retrieved May 24, 2009).

Mayo Clinic Staff. "Stroke: Treatment." July 3, 2008. www.mayoclinic.com/health/stroke treatment/BN00056 (retrieved May 24, 2009).

Mayo Clinic Staff. "Stroke Treatment: Carotid and Intracranial Stents." July 25, 2007. www.mayoclinic.com/health/stroke-treatment/BN00056 (retrieved May 24, 2009).

Mayo Clinic Staff. "Trichinosis: Causes. " February 1, 2008. www.mayoclinic.com/health/trichinosis/DS00689/DSECTION=causes (retrieved May 21, 2009).

McAbee, Gary. "Lessons Can be Learned from Malpractice Cases Involving Meningitis." *American Academy of Pediatrics APP News* 24, no. 4 (April 2004): 180–82.

McAbee, Gary N., Charles Deitschel, and Jan Berger. "Pediatric Medicolegal Education in the 21st Century." *Pediatrics* 117, no. 5 (May 2006): 1790.

McFarland, L., and P. Bernasconi. "*Saccharomyces boulardii*: A Review of an Innovative Biotherapeutic Agent." *Microbial Ecology in Health and Disease* 6, no. 4 (July 1993): 157–71.

McKinney's Consolidtated Laws of New York. 2000. New York: McKinney's

Medical Practice.com. "National Medical Practice Statistics." ExpertHub Network. 2009. www.medicalmalpractice.com/National-Medical-malpractice-Facts.cfm (retrieved March 3, 2009).

"Medicine's Dirty Little Secret: Hospitals Promote Doctors to Wash Their Hands." *Washington Post*, September 30, 1997.

Mehta, R. H., and K. A. Eagle. "Missed Diagnosis of Acute Coronary Syndromes in the Emergency Room: Continuing Challenges." *New England Journal of Medicine* 342 (April 2000): 1207–10.

Moore, Thomas J. "Time to Act on Drug Safety." *Journal of the American Medical Associations* 279 (May 1998): 1571.

Musgrove, Philip, Riadh Zeramdini, and Guy Carrin. "Basic Patterns in National Health Expenditures." *Bulletin of the World Health Organization* 80, no. 2 (February 2002): 134–42.

National Center for Health Statistics. National Vital Statistics System. www.cdc.gov/nchs/ nvss.htm (retrieved May 21, 2009).

National Institutes of Health. "Consensus Development Conference Statement: Cervical Cancer." *NIH Consensus Statement Online 1996 April 1–3*, 43, no. 1 (1996): 1–38. http:// consensus.nih.gov/1996/1996CervicalCancer102html.htm (retrieved May 24, 2009).

National Women's Law Center. "Nowhere to Turn." www.nwlc.org/archive. cfm?section=archive (retrieved April 8, 2009).

Newfield, James. "Current Issues in Providing Wound Care in the Home." *Home Health Care Management* 17, no. 3 (2005): 233–42.

News-Medical. "Cigna Reach Agreement on Physician Ranking System." October 30, 2007. www.newsmedical.net/print_article.asp?id=31931 (retrieved April 25, 2009).

Nuttall, Gregory A., Linda Stehling, Christopher Beighley, and Ronald J. Faust. "Current Transfusion Practices of Members of the American Society of Anesthesiologists: A Survey." *Anesthesiology* 99, no. 6 (December 2003): 1433–43.

Oldmixon, Seth. *Public Citizen Congress Watch 2007.* Washington, DC: Public Citizen's Congress Watch, 2007.

Pasley, Jessica. "Nursing Shortage Hurts Patients." *Vanderbilt Medical Center's Weekly Newspaper.* April 27, 2001. www.mc.vanderbilt.edu/reporter/index.html?ID=1480 (retrieved May 24, 2009).

Physicians' Financial News. "Doctors, Fearing Liability Suits, Resign." *Physicians' Financial News* (1997): 47.

Poulton, A. "Growth on Stimulant Medication: Clarifying the Confusion: A Review." *Archive of Disease in Childhood* 90, no. 8 (August 2005): 801–6.

Pradhan, Aruna D., JoAnn E. Manson, Jacques E. Rossouw, David S. Siscovick, Charles P. Mouton, Nader Rifai, Robert B. Wallace, Rebecca D. Jackson, Mary B. Pettinger, and Paul M. Ridker. "Inflammatory Biomarkers, Hormone Replacement Therapy, and Incident Coronary Heart Disease: Prospective Analysis From the Women's Health Initiative Observational Study." *Journal of the American Medical Association* 288, no. 8 (August 2002): 980–87.

Public Citizen Press Room. "Kentucky Doctors Not Facing a Medical Malpractice Insurance Crisis, Public Citizen Report Shows: Biggest Health Problem Is the 4.7 Percent of Kentucky Doctors Who Are Responsible for 50 Percent of Medical Malpractice Payouts to Injured Patients." February 4, 2004. www.citizen.org/pressroom/Release.cfm. ID=1640 (retrieved May 18, 2009).

Rabin, Roni Caryn. "Heart Stents Found as Effective as Bypass for Many Patients." *New York Times,* February 20, 2009.

Rabinowitz, Edward. "Low Health Literacy Hits Physicians Where It Hurts." *Physician's Money Digest*, June 4, 2008.

Reinhold, Robert. "Crisis in Emergency Rooms: More Symptoms than Cures." *New York Times*, July 28, 1988, p. 1A.

Reising, Deanna L., and Patricia N. Allen. "Protecting Yourself from Malpractice Claims." *American Nurse Today* 2, no. 2 (February 2007): 39–43.

Reynolds, R. A., J. A. Rizzo, and M. L. Gonzalez. "The Cost of Medical Professional Liability." *Journal of the American Medical Association* 257 (1987): 2776–81.

Rosenfeld, Harvey. *Silent Violence, Silent Death: A Consumer's Guide to the Medical Malpractice Epidemic*. Washington, DC: Essential Books, 1994.

Royal, S. A., G. A. Cloud, and W. M. Atchison. "Malpractice in Pediatric Radiology: A Survey in the United States and Canada." *Pediatric Radiology* 24, no. 7 (November 1994): 519–22.

Rubasmen, D. "Jumping to Conclusions: Costs, Patients, and Physicians." *Physicians Financial News*, February 2001.

Sage, Linda. "Managed Care Incentives Should Be Disclosed." *Bio-Medicine* 27 (January 1999) http://news.bio-medicine.org/medicine-news-2/Managed-Care-Incentives-Should-Be-Disclosed (retrieved April 29, 2009).

Sage, Linda. www.sage@medicine.wustl.edu (retrieved May 21, 2009).

Saul, Stephanie. "In Sour Economy, Some Scale Back on Medications." *New York Times*, October 21, 2008.

Scholten, Amy. "Human Papillomavirus Testing." Beth Israel Deaconess Medical Center. 2008. www.bidmc.org/YourHealth/MedicalProcedures.aspx?ChunkID=32308 (retrieved May 23, 2009).

Studdert, David M., Michelle M. Mello, Atul A. Gawande, Tejal K. Gandhi, Allen Kachalia, Catherine Yoon, Ann Louise Puopolo, and Troyen A. Brennan. "Claims, Errors, and Compensation Payments in Medical Malpractice Litigation." *New England Journal of Medicine* 354, no. 19 (May 2006): 2024–33.

Tartter, Paul Ian, David Pace, Mark Frost, and Jonine L. Bernstein. "Delay in Diagnosis of Breast Cancer." *Annals of Surgery* 229, no. 1 (January 1999): 91–96.

Terry, Elisa Elizabeth King. "Do Increasing Rates of Autism in California Let Vaccines Off the Hook?" Associated Content, January 9, 2008. www.associatedcontent.com/article/531079/do_increasing_rates_of_autism_in_california.html?cat=70 (retrieved May 24, 2009).

Thomas, Eric J., and Troyen A. Brennan. "Incidence and Types of Preventable Adverse Events in Elderly Patients: Population Based Review of Medical Records." *British Medicine Journal* 320 (March 2000): 741–44.

"Thoughts for Emergency Medical Technicians, Paramedics and Emergency Physicians." *Pediatrics* supplement 96 (1995): 199–210.

USA Today. "Study: Off Label Drugs Often Prescribed." *USA Today*, May 8, 2006.

U.S. Cancer Statistics Working Group. "United States Cancer Statistics: 1999–2005 Incidence and Mortality Web-based Report." Atlanta: Department of Health and Human Services, Centers for Disease Control and Prevention, and National Cancer Institute, 2009. www.cdc.gov/uscs (retrieved May 24, 2009).

U.S. Department of Justice. "Civil Bench and Jury Trials in State Courts." Civil Justice Data Brief Office of Justice Programs: 2205.

Voice for the Uninsured. "The Health Care Crisis: Overview of the American Medical Association: Reform Proposal." 2008. www.voicefortheuninsured.org/pdf/proposalover view.pdf (retrieved January 28, 2009).

Wenzel, Richard P., and Michael B. Edmond. "The Impact of Hospital Acquired Blood Stream Infection." *Centers for Disease Control Special Issue* 7, no. 2 (March–April 2001).

Williams, M., M. V. Williams, R. M. Parker, D. W. Baker, N. S. Panikh, K. Pitkin, W. C. Coates, and J. R. Nurses. "Inadequate Functional Literacy among Patients at Two Public Health Hospitals." *Journal of the American Medical Association* 274, no. 21 (1995).

Winerman, Lea. "The Uninsured in America." Online NewsHour, April 6, 2007. www.pbs. org/newshour/indepth_coverage/health/uninsured/whoaretheuninsured.html (retrieved May 24, 2009).

Women's Health USA. "Health Services Utilization: Hospitalization: 2005." U.S. Department of Health and Human Services Health Resources and Services Administration. 2008. http://mchb.hrsa.gov/whusa08/hsu/pages/306h.html (retrieved May 24, 2009).

World Bank. "Medical Malpractice Systems Around the Group: Examples from the U.S. Tort Liability System and the Sweden-No Fault System." Health, Nutrition and Population (HPN) Human Development Sector Unit Europe and Central Asia Region. http://194.84.38.65/files/esw_files/malpractice_systems_eng.pdf (retrieved May 24, 2009).

Zwillich, Todd. "Drug Errors Injure 1.5 Million Annually." WebMD, July 20, 2006. www .webmd.com/news/20060720/report-drug-errors-injure-millions (retrieved July 9, 2009).

INDEX

AAP. *See* American Academy of Pediatrics

abdominal examination, 34, 93–94

abdominal organ, ruptured, 76

abdominal pain, 90–93

ACE. *See* angiotensin-converting enzyme

ACOG. *See* The American College of Obstetricians and Gynecologists

ACS. *See* American Cancer Society

acute abdomen, 8, 91

ADD. *See* attention deficit disorder

address, forwarding, 48–49

ADHD. *See* attention deficit hyperactivity disorder

adolescents: depression, 141–42; mental health issues in, treating, 141–42; monitoring medication, 144; treating late (17-22 years of age), 142

Aetna, 15

AFP. *See* alphafetoprotein testing

alanine aminotransferase (ALT), 95

allergy, medication, 34, 67, 151

alphafetoprotein testing (AFP), 123

ALT. *See* alanine aminotransferase

ambulance, 74–78; insurance coverage, 166

American Academy of Pediatrics (AAP), 127

American Cancer Society (ACS), 110

The American College of Obstetricians and Gynecologists (ACOG), 117, 127

American Medical Association (AMA), 193

American Society of Anesthesiology, 46

ampicillin, 67

anemia, 52

anesthesia, intravenous, 153, 179

angioplasty, 103–104

angiotensin-converting enzyme (ACE), 105

antibiotics, 34; accepting, 168; children, use on, 57; diarrhea during/after taking, 80, 137–38,

184; infection and, 181; injudicious use of, 61; intravenous, 36, 49, 51; misuse of, 160–61, 169–70; oral v. intravenous, 40–41; prophylactic, 182–84; surgery, before, 181–82; symptoms and, 37; viral infections and, 135. *See also* prophylactic antibiotics

anticoagulation therapy, 184–85

antidepressants, 143; rapid reduction of, 144; suicide and, 142

antioxidants, 109

appendicitis, 35, 51; first signs of, 91

Archives of Internal Medicine, 40

ART. *See* assisted reproductive technologies

aspartate aminotransferase (AST), 94–95

assisted reproductive technologies (ART), 121–22

AST. *See* aspartate aminotransferase

atorvastatin, 19

attention deficit disorder (ADD), 140–41

attention deficit hyperactivity disorder (ADHD), 57–58, 63, 140–41

autism, 62, 65

Baby and Child Care (Spock), 64

backache, pregnancy, 124

bacterial infections, 133–34

bacteria mutation, 45, 61

behavioral pediatrics, 63

behavior disabilities, 140, 142–43. *See also* specific disabilities

Bell's palsy, 40

beta-blockers, 104–5

birth: defects, 123, 127–28; delivery, 59, 124; weight, 60. *See also* specific methods of delivery

blood: pressure, 30, 106, 118, 181; transfusion, 173. *See also* white blood cell counts

Board of Health of Westchester County, 60–61

Boren, James H., 177

Bornholm disease, 81–82

Bradley method, 124

brain tumor, secondary headaches and, 89

breast cancer, 111; chest pain and, 81–82; delay in diagnosis of, 170–71; HRT and, 127

breast examination, 118, 120

breast feeding, 59

bypass surgery versus stenting, 103–4

Caesarian sections. *See* C sections

calorie content in fast food, 61

cancer, 115; biopsy, 111–12; centers, 108, 198–99; diagnosis, 110–11; diagnostic tools for, 31; information resources, 214; nutrition and, 108–9; outpatient centers, 114; research, 109; second opinions, 112; staging of, 113. *See also* specific types of cancer

cancer therapy: alternative treatments, 114–15; approaches to, 113; business of, 114; choosing a doctor for, 110

cardiac catheterization, 85, 102, 104

cardiologists, 47

catastrophic coverage, 23

CBC. *See* completed blood cell count

Centers for Disease Control and Prevention, 160

cervical cancer, 119, 126

cervical dysplasia, 120

chemotherapy, 113–14, 199; side effects, 112

chest cancer, 172
chest pain, 81–84; diagnosis, 84–86
Chicago Tribune (2002), 161
child health care, 57, 192–93
children: antibiotics on, use of, 57;
    immunizations and, 62, 64; mental
    health issues in, treating, 140–41;
    multidisciplinary approach to, 63;
    obesity and, 61; second opinions
    and, 58; viral illness in, 61; white
    blood cell counts in, 58
chorionic villus sampling (CVS), 123
chronic mononucleosis, 46–47
Cigna Insurance Company, 15
Clinton, Hillary Rodham, 196
Clostridium difficile, 79–80, 137–38
Clostridium perfringens, 136
colonoscopy, 153
colposcopy, 120
comfort food, 61
communication: malpractice and,
    38–39; patient/doctor, 27–30
completed blood cell count (CBC), 84
computed tomography (CT), 90; ER,
    76, 78; insurance coverage and,
    15–16; smokers and, 175–76
conception, 122–25; folic acid and, 59
continuous fevers, 131
copay, 58
coronary artery disease, 83, 106–7;
    care for, 103; death by, 101;
    diagnosing, 86; gender and, 105;
    information resources on, 214–15;
    symptoms and treatments, 104–5;
    in young people, 102–3
cortisone, 130, 134, 153, 181–82
costochondritis, 82
coughs, 135
coxsackie B, 81–82
C-reactive protein, 105
C sections, 59, 125

CT. *See* computed tomography
cul-de-sac, 16; fluid in, 35
cultures, 36–37, 134, 138, 160–61
Cuomo, Andrew, 15
CVS. *See* chorionic villus sampling
cylindrical tubes. *See* stents versus
    bypass surgery

death, 201–2; by coronary artery
    disease, 101; due to physician error,
    39–40, 50; in ER, 77; health literacy
    and, 53; hospital rates, 161–62;
    preventable, rates, 191–92
demographic changes, 26–27; address
    updates, 48–50
Department of Justice (U.S.),
    malpractice trial data, 196–97
depression, 143; adolescents and,
    141–42; in geriatric age groups,
    143; pregnancy, 124–25; psychotic,
    143
developmental defects, 60
diagnosis: cultures for, 36–37; delay
    in, 76, 170–71; of fevers, 133–34;
    PCP, 34; treating for false, 46–47;
    understanding, 32, 53. *See also*
    second opinions
diarrhea: postantibiotic, 184; while
    taking antibiotics, 80, 137–38, 184
diet, 23, 25, 61
disequilibrium, 87–88
diverticulitis, 16, 79, 91, 94–95
dizziness, 86; disequilibrium, 87–88;
    vertigo, 87
doctor-patient relationship, 27–29,
    33, 51; communication, 27–30;
    hospitalists and, 74
doctor visits: follow-up, 152;
    preparation for, 29, 55; punctuality
    and behavior, 25–27; recording
    consultations, 54; routine

examination, 30; taking notes and asking questions, 29–30, 54–55
drug(s): computer entry systems, 68; injuries, 68; interactions, 68–71, 181–82; labels, 69. *See also* medication(s)

EBT. *See* examination before trial
ECT. *See* electroconvulsive therapy
electroconvulsive therapy (ECT), 139, 143
emergency room (ER), 73–74, 96–97; abdominal pain and, 90–93; avoiding, 95; checking into, 80–81; chest pains and, 81–86; closing of, 75; CT scan in, 76, 78; death in, 77; dizziness and, 86–88; examination, procedures, and tests, 93–96; fever and, 134; headaches, 88–90; overcrowded, 75, 77; physicians, 76; preparations, 78; presyncope and, 88; specialists in, 76–77
encephalopathy, 62
endocarditis, 37, 67
endocrine disorders, diagnostic tools for, 31
epidural hematoma, secondary headaches and, 89
ER. *See* emergency room
error(s): death due to physician, 39–40, 50; in ER, 75; eradication of, 44, 46; labeling, 173–74; medication, 68–69, 171; poor handwriting, 68–69
errors, admitting, 44, 195–96; insurance coverage and, 42; to physicians, 43
Escherichia coli (*E. coli*), 92, 137
esophageal ailments, 82
examination before trial (EBT), 48

fainting. *See* presyncope
family doctor. *See* pediatrician
fast food, 61
FDA. *See* Food and Drug Administration
fetal alcohol syndrome, 124
fever, 30, 130–31; causes of, 132–33; patterns in symptoms of, 131–32; postsurgery, 136; treating and diagnosing cause of, 133–34. *See also* specific fevers
Fixx, Jim, 17–18
folic acid, 59
Food and Drug Administration (FDA), 108
food poisoning, 136–37
From Anecdote to Antidote (Klein), 28

gallbladder, 95; attack, 82; stones, 91
gamma glutamyl transferase (GGT), 94–95
Gardasil, 125–26
gastritis, 82
gastroenterologist, 52
gastroesophageal reflux disease (GERD), 82
gastrointestinal bleeding, 52
general medical information resources, 213–14
genital warts, 119
GERD. *See* gastroesophageal reflux disease
geriatric age, treating mental health issues in, 143
GGT. *See* gamma glutamyl transferase
Goldwyn, Samuel, 157
Google, 41, 46, 63, 69
Gore, Albert, 1
Grasso, Benjamen, 144
gynecologist visits, 118–19, 143; annual, 117–18; first, 117

handwriting, poor, 68–70
headaches, 88; primary headaches,
    88–89; secondary headaches, 89–90
health care: ads against universal, 19;
    participation in, 8–10; U.S., 191–95.
    See also child health care; general
    medicine information resources;
    managed health care programs;
    preventative health care; universal
    health care
HealthGrades, Inc., 159–60, 180,
    202; Hospital Quality Study, 11th
    annual, 161–62; Patient Safety in
    American Hospitals Study, 162–63,
    204n3
health literacy, 53
health maintenance, 30
health maintenance organizations
    (HMO), 15–16, 194
heart attack, 75, 103; hereditary factors
    of, 17–18; missing diagnosis of, 76;
    procedures following, 104
heart disease. *See* coronary artery
    disease
Heart Outcomes Prevention
    Evaluation (HOPE), 208n8
Helicobacter pylori, 95
hepatobiliary iminodiacetic acid
    (HIDA) scanning, 95
hernia, 91
herpes zoster, 81, 180
HIDA. *See* hepatobiliary iminodiacetic
    acid scanning
HMO. *See* health maintenance
    organizations
Hodgkin's disease, 112–13
HOPE. *See* Heart Outcomes
    Prevention Evaluation
hormone replacement therapy (HRT),
    126–27
Hospital Compare, 180

hospitalist, 74
Hospital Quality Study, 11th annual,
    161–62
hospitals, 108, 158, 166–68; for
    baby delivery, choosing, 59, 124;
    cancer outpatient centers, 114;
    checking in, 164–65; death rates
    and quality study, 161–62; falling
    in, 163; information resources, 214;
    insurance coverage and, 15, 150;
    malpractice in, 158–61; medication
    during, stays, 9; patient safety
    studies, 162–63; staff, 161; teaching,
    cutbacks, 21. *See also* emergency
    room
HPV. *See* human papillomavirus
HRT. *See* hormone replacement
    therapy
human papillomavirus (HPV), 118;
    types of, 119; vaccinations, 125–26
Hunter, James, M., 169
hygiene, 26

IgG. *See* immunoglobulin G
IgM. *See* immunoglobulin M
immunizations, 57; children and, 62,
    64. *See also* vaccines
immunoglobulin G (IgG), 64
immunoglobulin M (IgM), 64
infection, 36, 64; antibiotics and, 181;
    clostridial, 80; cross-infection, 167;
    delayed treatment for, 38, 49, 67;
    as leading cause of malpractice,
    159–60; limiting susceptibility
    to, 167; local, 129; of lungs, 83;
    neurologic, 136; respiratory, 135;
    staph, 199; surgeons, rate by, 44–
    45; surgery, post, 31, 44–45, 129,
    150, 199; surgery, prior to, 180;
    white blood count and, 35. *See
    also* bacterial infections; infectious

disease; systemic infections; viral
   infections
infectious disease, 49, 129, 138;
   consultations, 51; treating, 130
infertility, 120–22
influenza, 135
The Institute for Syphilis and
   Dermatology, 41
Institute of Medicine (IOM), 67, 77,
   159, 160
insurance, 107–8, 165, 191;
   ambulance, 166; applicants, 14;
   approval/permission from, 15–18;
   catastrophic coverage, 23; CT and
   MRI, 15–16; discrimination and,
   20; from employers, 23; errors,
   admitting, and, 42; hospitalization
   and, 15, 150; information resources,
   214; maternity care, 20; medication,
   19, 108; money spent, 194–95;
   obtaining for the uninsured, 193;
   policies and profits, 13–20, 23;
   protection, 23; refusals, 204n7;
   secondary, 22; types of, 10–11, 22.
   See also malpractice insurance;
   Medicare
insurance companies, 193; medical
   staffs of, 18. See also specific
   companies
intermittent fevers, 131
intestinal parasites, 92
intravenous line, 167
in vitro fertilization (IVF), 121–22
IOM. See Institute of Medicine
IVF. See in vitro fertilization

Joint Commission of Hospitals, 108

Kerry, John, 191
kidney stones, 91
Klein, Richard S., 28

Kocher, Gerhard, 7
Kucinich, Dennis, 193, 195

labeling, 175; FDA, 108; improper, 55;
   laboratory errors, 173–74; second
   opinions, 175
laboratory, 172–75; avoiding errors,
   176; identification errors, 173–74;
   testing, 94
language, simple, 53–54
lawsuits, malpractice, 195–97;
   frivolous, 197
lawyer: fees, 198; quality of, 42–43
LDL. See low-density lipoprotein
learning disabilities, 140
leukemia, 46–47
lithium, 142
Los Angeles Times (2008), 126
low-density lipoprotein (LDL), 105
lung cancer, 18, 171–72, 176
lungs, disease of, 82–83
Lyme arthritis, 36, 49
Lyme disease, 39–41, 48, 63; chest
   pain and, 81–82

magnetic resonance images (MRI),
   89–90; insurance coverage and,
   15–16
"Making Patient Safety the
   Centerpiece of Medical Liability
   Reform" (Clinton & Obama), 196
malpractice, 201; alterations of
   records and, 43–44; causes of, 158,
   161; communication and, 38–39;
   contract, 42; in hospitals, 158–61;
   leading causes of, 32, 68, 159–60;
   limits on, claims, 40; office, 40;
   payouts, 210–11n3; in psychiatry,
   144; recommendations to prevent,
   160; statistics, 1–2, 46, 159–60;
   suspecting, 47; trial data from U.S.

Department of Justice, 196–97;
uninsured and, 193–94. *See also*
errors, admitting
malpractice cases, 171; examples of,
34–39, 78–80, 102, 129–30, 165,
201–2; in Kentucky, 210–11n3;
prospective physicians and past,
33–34; reviews, 198–201
malpractice insurance, 10, 42, 194;
lawsuits and, 195–97; rates, 196,
198
mammogram, 111, 120; second
opinions, 175
managed health care programs, 74
mania, 142
manic depressive behavior, 142–43
maternity care, 20
McQueen, Steve, 108, 115
M. D. *See Medicinea Doctor*
medical education, 44
medical injuries, office, 43
medical school class rankings, 50
medical staffs, insurance companies, 18
medical terms, 53
Medicare, 21–22, 194, 205n15; patient
records, 161–62
medication(s): adolescents on,
monitoring, 144; allergies to, 34, 67,
151; antimanic, 142; biases towards,
140; errors, 68–69, 71; fevers within
24 hours of taking, 132; during
hospital stays, 9; insurance coverage
and, 19, 108; maintaining lists of,
70; mental health, 139–40, 144;
necessity of prescribed, 54–56, 71;
personal histories of, 92; surgery,
interactions before, 181–82. *See
also* antibiotics; drug(s); general
medical information resources;
psychiatric medicines
medicine, organized, 197–202

Medicinea Doctor (M. D.), 139
Mencken, Henry Louis, 129
meningitis, 45
menstrual cycle, 35, 117
mental health, 145; adolescents,
treating, 141–42; children, treating,
140–41; geriatric age group,
treating, 143; late adolescents (17-
22), treating, 142; medication and,
139–40, 144; middle years, treating,
142–43. *See also* specific illnesses
meperidine, 8
methicillin-resistant *Staphylococcus
aureus* (MRSA), 61
methylphenidate, 58, 141
miscarriage, 123
mononucleosis test, 34
Moore, Michael, 14
motor vehicle accidents, 48, 74
MRI. *See* magnetic resonance images
multidisciplinary approach, 63
murmurs, 83–84

narcotics, 8
The National Cancer Center, 108
National Cancer Institute (NCI), 109
National Data Bank, 33
National Registry, 55
National Women's Law Center, 20
Navigator Program, 110
NCI. *See* National Cancer Institute
neonatal: intensive care, 59; mortality,
60
neonatology, 60
neurologic infection, 136
New England Journal of Medicine, 126
New York Times, 20, 40
nursing homes, 73

Obama, Barack, 196
obesity, 60–61

obstetrics, controversies in, 125–26
oncologist, 108, 114
Ordent, Michel, 124
osteomyelitis, 38
outpatient: facilities, 114, 150–51;
    procedure, 151–52, 168
ovarian follicle, ruptured, 35

PA. See physician's assistant
pacemakers, 105–6
pain, acute, 76
pancreatic diseases, 95
Papanicolaou, George, 118
Pap smears, 117–18; abnormal, 119;
    frequency of, 118–19
parenthood, rules to follow, 59
patient(s), 108–9; falling, 163; fear in,
    28–29; Medicare records, 161–62;
    pediatric, 60; per nurse ratios,
    161, 168; preoperative, 167; rights,
    fighting for, 197–202; safety studies,
    162–63, 204n3; welfare, 74. See
    also doctor-patient relationship;
    outpatient
Patient Safety in American Hospitals
    Study, 162–63, 204n3
PCP. See primary care physician
pediatrician, 57, 65; choosing, 58–59;
    interviews, 59; routine visits, 59
pediatric patients, 60
pediatric surgeon, 65
pericarditis, 83
pharmaceutical companies, 69
pharmacists, 68
physical examination, by organ system,
    31–32
physician: choosing, 50–51; choosing
    the wrong, 51–52; competency
    of, 111; costs for, 74; ER, 76;
    handwriting, 68–69; prospective,
    33–34; recommendations, 51;

"report card," 46, 55; review,
    47. See also doctor-patient
    relationship; pediatrician; primary
    care physician
physician error: admitting, 40; deaths
    due to, 39–40, 50; denying, 41–42
physician's assistant (PA), 67
Physicians' Desk Reference, 163
pleurisy, 82–83
postmenopausal bleeding, 117
pregnancy, 122–25, 128; backache,
    124; depression and postpartum
    depression, 124–25; early signs
    of, 124; evaluations, 122–23; first
    trimester screen, 123; smoking and
    drinking during, 124; weight-related
    problems during, 123–24. See also
    birth
prenatal care, 59, 123; testing, 122
prescription(s): coverage, 22–23;
    incorrect filling of, 68; legibility of,
    68–70; wrong, 67–68
presyncope, 88
preventative health care, 21
primary care physician (PCP):
    diagnosis and treatment plan,
    34; obtaining patient test results,
    47–48; referral, 15
proactive practice, 51, 68, 70; ER
    and, 95
probiotics, 184
prophylactic antibiotics, 182–84
prostate biopsy, 37
psychiatric medicines, 139–40, 143;
    side effects, 144. See also specific
    medicines
psychiatrists, 58, 139–40; malpractice
    among, 144
psychoanalysis, 139–40
psychologists, 139–40
psychotherapy, 139

pulmonary embolism, 83
pulse, 30

questions, asking, 29–30, 54–55;
   before surgery, 179–80; importance
   of, 52–55; open-ended v. closed-
   ended, 31; undressed, 54

radiation therapy, 109
radiology, 170–72; second opinions,
   175
records, alterations of, 43–44
rectal bleeding, 91
rectal examination, 94
referrals, 16–17, 50
reimbursement rates, 14–15; shortages
   and, 77
remittent fever, 132
reproductive endocrinologists, 120–21
respiration rate, 30
respiratory infections, 135
rib pain, 82
Ritalin. *See* methylphenidate
Rosenfeld, Harvey, 1
routine examination, 30

Saccharomyces boulardii, 184
Salmonella, 136–37
schizophrenia, 142
screen testing, 111
second opinions, 35–36, 54, 56, 63,
   154, 166, 175, 179, 198–99; cancer
   and, 112; children and, 58; for
   senior citizens, 36
senior citizens: Medicare and, 21;
   second opinions for, 36. *See also*
   geriatric age, treating mental health
   issues in
sexual intercourse, bleeding post, 117
sexually transmitted diseases (STDs),
   117; testing, 118

shaking chills, severe, 131
Shigella, 137
shock therapy. *See* electroconvulsive
   therapy
Sicko, 14
side effects, 69, 71; of anitmanic
   medications, 142; chemotherapy,
   112; of psychiatric medicines, 144
SIDS. *See* sudden infant death
   syndrome
Simms, Sy, 9, 41
simvastatin (Zocor), 19
smokers, 175–76
specialists, 14–15; choosing, 51; in
   ER, 76–77; fertility, 121; growing
   numbers, 74–75
sperm evaluation, 121
spirochete, 41
Spock, Benjamin, 64
Staphylococcus, 130, 136
State Professional Licensing Bureau, 33
statins, 105–6
STD. *See* sexually transmitted diseases
stents versus bypass surgery, 103–4
stimulants, 141
stress, 25; echocardiograms, 101–2
stress tests, 52, 84; approvals for, 17–
   18; inaccuracies of, 101
stroke: information resources on, 214–
   15; secondary headaches and, 89
subdural hematomas, secondary
   headaches and, 89
sudden infant death syndrome (SIDS),
   124
suicide, 142
supplements, 108–9
supraclavicular lymph node
   enlargements, 171–72
surgery, 154–55; after, 186–87;
   antibiotics and drug interactions
   before, 181–82; anticoagulation

therapy, 184–85; deciding
on, 177–79; environment, 45;
exploratory, 34–35; fevers post,
136; gynecological, 43; without
hospitalization, 150; infections
and, 31, 44–45, 129, 150, 180,
199; outpatient, 151–52, 168; prior
to, 180–81, 185–86; prophylactic
antibiotics and, 183; questions
before, 179–80
symptoms: antibiotic and, 37; cardiac,
52; coronary artery disease,
104–5; with fever, 131–32; of food
poisoning, 136–37; overplaying, 75,
80; of pregnancy, 124; progression
of, 92; requiring medical care, 63
syphilis, 41
systemic infections, 129–30

Tagore, Rabindranath, 57
taxpayers, 21
telephone number, forwarding, 48
test results, 38–39; obtaining copies of,
32–33, 47–48, 56, 170; overlooking
abnormal, 39
therapists: choosing, 140, 145; M. D.-
trained v. non-M. D., 139–40
therapy, talk, 140, 143
three Q program, 63
Tjarkovsky, Igor, 124
treatment, delayed, 38, 49, 67
treatment plan, 35–36; dialogue for
effective, 33; PCP, 34
Trichinosis, 137
Turley, Roul, 13

ulcer disease, 82
ultrasound, 82
uninsured, 74, 75; insurance, obtaining
for, 193; malpractice and, 193–94

United States (U.S.): government
debt, 21–22; health care system,
191–95; malpractice statistics,
159–60; neonatal mortality,
ranking for, 60; ranking by WHO,
60, 107
universal health care, 19, 60, 68–69,
108, 193, 195
University of Rome, 41
urinary catheters, 167
U.S. See United States
USA Today, 55

vaccines, 125–26; reactions to,
possible, 62. See also immunizations
vertigo, 87
Viagra, 182
violence, 74
viral illness, 61
viral infections, 133–34; antibiotics
and, 135
vitamins: A, 59; C, 59; cancer patients
and, 108–9; D, 59; prenatal, 123

Walton, Bill, 149
weight fluctuations, 30, 31
weight gain, 31; during pregnancy,
123–24
welfare patients, 74
white blood cell counts, 35, 84, 134,
173; in children, 58
WHO. See World Health Organization
women: health, 117–20; infertility,
121; insurance and, 20
World Health Organization (WHO),
191; ratings, 13–14; U.S. rankings,
60, 107

x-rays: annual, 172; obtaining copies,
175

ABOUT THE AUTHOR

The art of medicine consists in amusing the patient while nature cures the disease."

~ Voltaire

Richard S. Klein, M.D. is a practicing physician in Yorktown Heights, New York. He specializes in internal medicine and infectious diseases. An associate professor of medicine, Dr. Klein teaches medical students at the New York Medical College.

An internationally renowned caregiver, Dr. Klein has been knighted by the Italian government and received medals and awards from the Israeli government. As a young sailor, he was awarded many lifesaving commendations for his work as a field medic.

He ran for U.S. Congress from the New York 19th Congressional District. At that time he met the president and vice-president of the United States, as well as most Democratic representatives and senators. He has had two private audiences with the late Pope John Paul II. He has also met with all the major leaders of Israel since 1967.

Dr. Klein was the Westchester county chairman of Israeli Bonds and the UJA-Federation. He presently serves on the boards of a multitude of volunteer organizations, serving the community as both physician and volunteer. Dr. Klein is the author of *The Wine Tasters Album*. He also founded the Drs. Fast diet system. An instrument rated aircraft pilot and a second degree black belt in karate, Dr. Klein has sailed his '47 Choy Lee, *DRSFAST*, all around the east coast of the United States, as well as throughout the Caribbean.

Dr. Klein has recently been appointed to serve on the Board of the Department of Health of Westchester County.

Dr. Klein lives with his wife, Caryn, twelve-year-old stepdaughter, Arianna, and three-year-old son, Matthew, in Somers, New York. He also has two adult daughters (Elyse and Jessica).

Dr. Klein's first book, *From Anecdote to Antidote*, was released in June 2008.

Al Roker, of the Today Show, said, "Dr. Klein has the perfect antidote for the usual boring medical memoir."

Robert F. Kennedy, Jr. said, "Dr. Klein's experiences and his knack for solving medical mysteries aren't just fun to read, they inspire readers to listen to their bodies and trust their instincts, two keys to remaining healthy and happy."